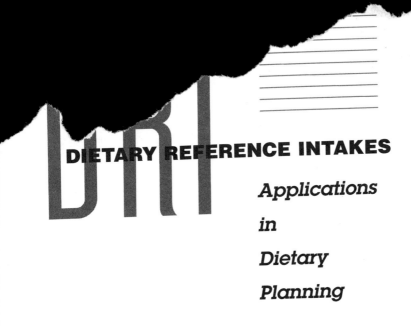

DIETARY REFERENCE INTAKES

Applications

in

Dietary

Planning

Subcommittee on Interpretation and Uses of
Dietary Reference Intakes
and the
Standing Committee on the Scientific Evaluation of
Dietary Reference Intakes

INSTITUTE OF MEDICINE
OF THE NATIONAL ACADEMIES

THE NATIONAL ACADEMIES PRESS
Washington, D.C.
www.nap.edu

IE NATIONAL ACADEM

NOTICE: The project that is the subject of
of the National Research Council, whose m
National Academy of Sciences, the National Academy of
Medicine. The members of the committee responsible for the
special competences and with regard for appropriate balance.

Support for this project was provided by the U.S. Department of Agriculture, Economic Research Service, Contract No. 43-3AEM-1-80053; Health Canada; U.S. Department of Health and Human Services, Office of Disease Prevention and Health Promotion, Contract No. 282-96-0033; Dannon Institute; and the Dietary Reference Intakes Corporate Donors' Fund. Contributors to the Fund include Roche Vitamins Inc., Mead Johnson Nutritionals, and M&M/Mars. The opinions or conclusions expressed herein are those of the Subcommittee on Interpretation and Uses of Dietary Reference Intakes and are not necessarily those of the funding organizations.

Library of Congress Cataloging-in-Publication Data

Dietary reference intakes : applications in dietary planning /
Subcommittee on Interpretation and Uses of Dietary Reference Intakes and
the Standing Committee on the Scientific Evaluation of Dietary Reference
Intakes.
      p. ; cm.
Includes bibliographical references and index.
  ISBN 0-309-08714-7 (hardcover : alk. paper) – ISBN 0-309-08853-4
(pbk. : alk. paper)
  1. Nutrition. 2. Reference values (Medicine)
  [DNLM: 1. Nutrition Assessment. 2. Energy Intake. 3. Nutrition
Policy. 4. Nutritional Requirements. 5. Reference Standards. QU 146
D5658 2003] I. Institute of Medicine (U.S.). Subcommittee on
Interpretation and Uses of Dietary Reference Intakes. II. Institute of
Medicine (U.S.). Standing Committee on the Scientific Evaluation of
Dietary Reference Intakes.
  QP141.D527 2003
  613.2–dc21

                        2003006783

ISBN 0-309-51882-2 (PDF)

This report is available from the National Academies Press, 500 Fifth Street, N.W., Lockbox 285, Washington, DC 20055; (800) 624-6242 or (202) 334-3313 (in the Washington metropolitan area); Internet, http://www.nap.edu.

For more information about the Institute of Medicine, visit the IOM home page at: **www.iom.edu.**

The serpent has been a symbol of long life, healing, and knowledge among almost all cultures and religions since the beginning of recorded history. The serpent adopted as a logotype by the Institute of Medicine is a relief carving from ancient Greece, now held by the Staatliche Museen in Berlin.

"Knowing is not enough; we must apply.
Willing is not enough; we must do."
—Goethe

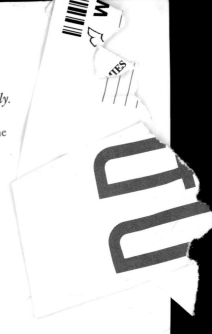

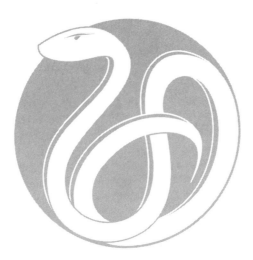

INSTITUTE OF MEDICINE
OF THE NATIONAL ACADEMIES

Shaping the Future for Health

THE NATIONAL ACADEMIES
Advisers to the Nation on Science, Engineering, and Medicine

The **National Academy of Sciences** is a private, nonprofit, self-perpetuating society of distinguished scholars engaged in scientific and engineering research, dedicated to the furtherance of science and technology and to their use for the general welfare. Upon the authority of the charter granted to it by the Congress in 1863, the Academy has a mandate that requires it to advise the federal government on scientific and technical matters. Dr. Bruce M. Alberts is president of the National Academy of Sciences.

The **National Academy of Engineering** was established in 1964, under the charter of the National Academy of Sciences, as a parallel organization of outstanding engineers. It is autonomous in its administration and in the selection of its members, sharing with the National Academy of Sciences the responsibility for advising the federal government. The National Academy of Engineering also sponsors engineering programs aimed at meeting national needs, encourages education and research, and recognizes the superior achievements of engineers. Dr. Wm. A. Wulf is president of the National Academy of Engineering.

The **Institute of Medicine** was established in 1970 by the National Academy of Sciences to secure the services of eminent members of appropriate professions in the examination of policy matters pertaining to the health of the public. The Institute acts under the responsibility given to the National Academy of Sciences by its congressional charter to be an adviser to the federal government and, upon its own initiative, to identify issues of medical care, research, and education. Dr. Harvey V. Fineberg is president of the Institute of Medicine.

The **National Research Council** was organized by the National Academy of Sciences in 1916 to associate the broad community of science and technology with the Academy's purposes of furthering knowledge and advising the federal government. Functioning in accordance with general policies determined by the Academy, the Council has become the principal operating agency of both the National Academy of Sciences and the National Academy of Engineering in providing services to the government, the public, and the scientific and engineering communities. The Council is administered jointly by both Academies and the Institute of Medicine. Dr. Bruce M. Alberts and Dr. Wm. A. Wulf are chair and vice chair, respectively, of the National Research Council.

www.national-academies.org

v

Staff

ALLISON A. YATES, Study Director
MARY POOS, Senior Program Officer
PAULA TRUMBO, Senior Program Officer
GAIL E. SPEARS, Staff Editor
SANDRA AMAMOO-KAKRA, Senior Project Assistant

Preface

This report is the second of a series intended to provide guidance in using Dietary Reference Intakes (DRIs). Its focus is the applications of DRIs in dietary planning. This report, and the previous report in this series on applicaiton of DRIs in dietary assessment, is from the Subcommittee on Interpretation and Uses of Dietary Reference Intakes (Uses Subcommittee) of the Standing Committee on the Scientific Evaluation of Dietary Reference Intakes (DRI Committee).

The Food and Nutrition Board anticipated that substantive guidance would be needed by U.S. and Canadian health professionals in the transition to the new DRIs developed jointly by Canadian and American scientists. These new values represent a significant departure from the former Recommended Dietary Allowances (RDAs) for the United States and Recommended Nutrient Intakes (RNIs) for Canada.

In the past, RDAs and RNIs were the primary values available to U.S. and Canadian health professionals for planning and assessing the diets of individuals and groups. The new DRIs represent a more complete set of values. They were developed in recognition of the growing and diverse uses of quantitative reference values and the availability of more sophisticated approaches for dietary planning and assessment purposes. The Uses Subcommittee approached its work in two phases; this report examines the appropriate use of each type of available DRI value in planning nutrient intakes of groups and individuals. The earlier report presented information on the appropriate uses of specific DRI values in assessing diets for groups and individuals. Each report reviews the statistical underpinnings for the various uses of the DRI values, illustrates these uses through sample applications, and provides guidelines to help professionals determine when specific uses are appropriate or inappropriate.

The Uses Subcommittee was charged to review the scientific literature regarding the uses of dietary reference standards and their applications, and to (1) provide guidance for the appropriate applications of DRIs for specific purposes, (2) identify inappropriate applications of these values, (3) evaluate various assumptions regarding intake and requirement distributions, (4) review adjustments needed to minimize potential errors in dietary intake data, and (5) give special consideration, as appropriate, to the uses of DRI values of specific nutrients. A brief description of the overall DRI project is given in Appendix A.

This report has been reviewed in draft form by individuals chosen for their diverse perspectives and technical expertise, in accordance with procedures approved by the NRC's Report Review Committee. The purpose of this independent review is to provide candid and critical comments that will assist the institution in making its published report as sound as possible and to ensure that the report meets institutional standards for objectivity, evidence, and responsiveness to the study charge. The review comments and draft manuscript remain confidential to protect the integrity of the deliberative process. We wish to thank the following individuals for their review of this report:

Mikel Aickin, Kaiser Permanente Northwest Division; Phyllis E. Bowen, University of Illinois at Chicago; Helen H. Jensen, Iowa State University; Susan Krebs-Smith, National Cancer Institute; Mary J. Kretsch, University of California, Davis; George McCabe, Purdue University; Grace Ostenso, Washington, D.C.; Beatrice L. Rogers, Tufts University; and Christopher Sempos, SUNY Buffalo.

Although the reviewers listed above have provided many constructive comments and suggestions, they were not asked to endorse the conclusions or recommendations nor did they see the final draft of the report before its release. The review of this report was overseen by Eileen Kennedy, International Life Sciences Institute, and Enriqueta Bond, Burroughs Wellcome Fund. Appointed by the National Research Council and the Institute of Medicine, they were responsible for making certain that an independent examination of this report was carried out in accordance with institutional procedures and that all review comments were carefully considered. Responsibility for the final content of this report rests entirely with the authoring committee and the institution.

The support of the government of Canada in establishing the Uses Subcommittee represents an important component of a pioneering first step in the standardization of nutrient reference intakes in North America. The Canadian government's support of these activities and the participation of Canadian scientists as full partners in this effort are gratefully acknowledged.

The DRI Committee wishes to acknowledge, in particular, the commitment and dedication shown by Susan I. Barr who assumed the chairmanship of the Uses Subcommittee following completion of the first report on dietary assessment. Dr. Barr has steered this project through some very controversial issues to provide health professionals specific guidance on the appropriate use of these new dietary reference intake values for diet planning.

Sincere thanks are also extended to George H. Beaton, technical consultant to the DRI Committee, for his willingness to critically review this report during many phases of development. His thoughtful comments and constructive assistance provided an important impetus to move the conceptual framework forward during the project's developmental and subsequent stages. Not all issues have been resolved, but the foundation for addressing them has been strengthened significantly. We also extend special thanks to the staff of the Food and Nutrition Board and especially to Mary Poos, study director for the Uses Subcommittee, for her contributions to the synthesis of the report. We recognize that significant efforts were required by the Subcommittee and Food and Nutrition Board staff to complete the report. Thus on behalf of the DRI Committee and the Food and Nutrition Board, we wish to thank Allison A. Yates, Director of the Food and Nutrition Board and study director for the DRI activity, for her continued oversight, and also recognize, with appreciation, the contributions of Shelley Goldberg, Sybil Boggis, Harleen Sethi, Alice Vorosmarti, Leslie Vogelsang, and Paula Trumbo. We wish also to thank Gail Spears for editing the manuscript.

Cutberto Garza
Chair, Food and Nutrition Board

Contents

xiii

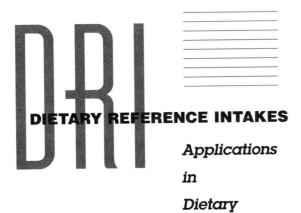

DIETARY REFERENCE INTAKES

Applications

in

Dietary

Planning

Summary

This report is the second of a series intended to provide guidance on the interpretation and uses of Dietary Reference Intakes (DRIs). The term *Dietary Reference Intakes* refers to a set of at least four nutrient-based reference values that can be used for assessing and planning diets and for many other purposes. Specifically, this report provides guidance to nutrition and health professionals for applications of the DRIs in dietary planning for individuals and groups, as well as providing the theoretical background and statistical justification for these applications.

A previous report examined the use of the DRIs in dietary assessment (IOM, 2000a). Dietary assessment using the DRIs, whether for individuals or groups, involves a comparison of usual nutrient intakes with nutrient requirements and examines the probability of inadequate or excessive intake.

Dietary planning, on the other hand, aims to optimize the prevalence of diets that are nutritionally adequate without being excessive. Dietary planning may be done at several different levels. It may refer to an individual planning a meal and food purchases, a food service manager in an institution planning food acquisition and menus, or a government agency planning large nutrition-related or food assistance programs. For the purposes of this report, dietary planning applies to planning intakes, rather than the amount of food purchased or served. Throughout this report methods for planning nutrient intakes of individuals and methods for planning nutrient intakes of groups are distinguished, as these are two very different applications.

1

Some of the dietary planning activities most relevant to use of the DRIs include individual dietary planning, dietary guidance, institutional food planning, military food and nutrition planning, planning for food assistance programs, food labeling, food fortification, developing new or modified food products, and assuring food safety. This document presents a framework for how the DRIs should be used and interpreted for these purposes.

WHAT ARE DIETARY REFERENCE INTAKES?

The *Dietary Reference Intakes* (DRIs) are a set of nutrient-based reference values that expand upon and replace the former Recommended Dietary Allowances (RDAs) in the United States and the Recommended Nutrient Intakes (RNIs) in Canada. The new DRIs differ from the former RDAs and RNIs conceptually in that (1) where specific data on safety and efficacy exist, reduction in the risk of chronic degenerative disease is included in the formulation of the recommendation rather than just the absence of signs of deficiency, (2) the concepts of probability and risk explicitly underpin the determination of the DRIs and inform their application in assessment and planning, (3) upper levels of intake are established where data exist regarding risk of adverse health effects, and (4) components of food that may not meet the traditional concept of a nutrient but are of possible benefit to health are reviewed, and if sufficient data exist, reference intakes are established.

A nutrient has either an Estimated Average Requirement (EAR) and an RDA, or an Adequate Intake (AI). When an EAR for the nutrient cannot be determined (and therefore, neither can the RDA), then an AI is established. In addition, many nutrients have a Tolerable Upper Intake Level (UL). A brief definition of each of the DRIs is presented in Box S-1.

An important principle underlying the former RDAs and RNIs, as well as the new DRIs, is that these are standards for apparently healthy people—not values that are meant to be applied to those with acute or chronic disease or for repletion of previously deficient individuals.

The chosen criterion of nutritional adequacy or adverse effect is different for each nutrient and is identified in the DRI nutrient reports (IOM, 1997, 1998a, 2000b, 2001, 2002a). Requirements are typically presented as a single number for various life stage and gender groups rather than as multiple endpoints except in the case of vitamin A. A more detailed discussion of the origin and framework of the DRIs is presented in Appendix A. Recommended in-

---

BOX S-1 Dietary Reference Intakes

Estimated Average Requirement (EAR): the average daily nutrient intake level estimated to meet the requirement of half the healthy individuals in a particular life stage and gender group.

Recommended Dietary Allowance (RDA): the average daily nutrient intake level sufficient to meet the nutrient requirement of nearly all (97 to 98 percent) healthy individuals in a particular life stage and gender group.

Adequate Intake (AI): a recommended average daily nutrient intake level based on observed or experimentally determined approximations or estimates of nutrient intake by a group (or groups) of healthy people that are assumed to be adequate—used when an RDA cannot be determined.

Tolerable Upper Intake Level (UL): the highest average daily nutrient intake level likely to pose no risk of adverse health effects to almost all individuals in a particular life stage and gender group. As intake increases above the UL, the potential risk of adverse health effects increases.

---

takes for the nutrients examined to date are presented at the end of this book.

Box S-2 provides a brief introduction to appropriate uses of the DRIs for planning.

IMPLEMENTATION OF DIETARY PLANNING FOR INDIVIDUALS AND GROUPS

Regardless of whether diets are being planned for individuals or for groups, the goal is to plan usual diets that are nutritionally adequate, or stated another way, such that the probability of nutrient inadequacy or excess is acceptably low. For individuals, the goal of planning is to achieve usual intakes that are close to the Recommended Dietary Allowance or the Adequate Intake (AI). For groups, the goal of planning is to determine a usual intake *distribution* that results in a low prevalence of intakes that are inadequate or at risk of being excessive. The Estimated Average Requirement, AI, and Tolerable Upper Intake Level are used in planning the diets of groups.

Figure S-1 schematically shows the various steps involved in implementing dietary plans for individuals and groups. Details of each step are discussed below.

BOX S-2 Uses of DRIs for Planning Intakes of Apparently Healthy Individuals and Groups

For an Individual

EAR[a]: should not be used as an intake goal for the individual.

RDA: plan for this intake; usual intake at or above this level has a low probability of inadequacy.

AI: plan for this intake; usual intake at or above this level has a low probability of inadequacy.

UL: plan for usual intake below this level to avoid potential risk of adverse effects from excessive nutrient intake.

For a Group

EAR[a]: use to plan for an acceptably low prevalence of inadequate intakes within a group.

RDA: should not be used to plan intakes of groups.

AI[b]: plan for mean intake at this level; mean usual intake at or above this level implies a low prevalence of inadequate intakes.

UL: use in planning to minimize the proportion of the population at potential risk of excessive nutrient intake.

[a]In the case of energy, an EER is provided. The EER is the dietary energy intake that is predicted (with variance) to maintain energy balance in a healthy adult of a defined age, gender, weight, height, and level of physical activity. In children and pregnant and lactating women, the EER includes the needs associated with deposition of tissues or secretion of milk at rates consistent with good health. For individuals, the EER represents the midpoint of a range within which an individual's energy requirements are likely to vary. As such, it is below the needs of half the individuals with the specified characteristics, and exceeds the needs of the other half. Body weight should be monitored and energy intake adjusted accordingly.

[b]The AI should be used with less confidence if it has not been established as a mean intake of a healthy group.

USING DIETARY REFERENCE INTAKES TO PLAN DIETS FOR INDIVIDUALS

Planning diets for individuals involves two steps. First, appropriate nutrient goals should be set, and second, a dietary plan that the individual will consume must be developed. This is most frequently accomplished using food-based guidance systems.

5

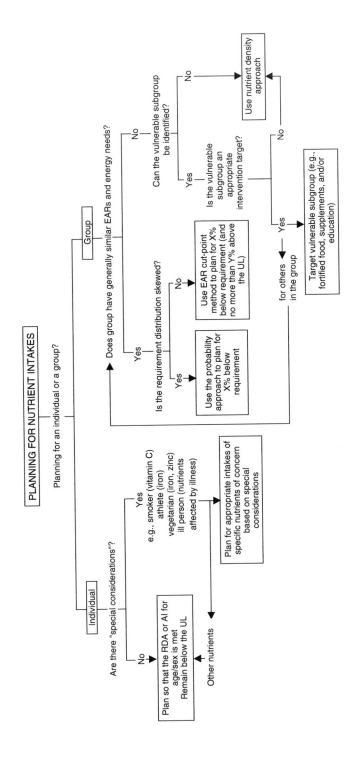

FIGURE S-1 Schematic decision tree for dietary planning.

Setting the Goal

The goal for individual planning is to ensure that the diet *as eaten* has an acceptably low risk of nutrient inadequacy while simultaneously minimizing the risk of nutrient excess for all nutrients for which Dietary Reference Intakes (DRIs) have been established. When planning for individuals for nutrients such as vitamins, minerals, and protein, a low risk of inadequacy is planned by meeting the Recommended Dietary Allowance (RDA) or Adequate Intake (AI), and a low risk of excess by remaining below the Tolerable Upper Intake Level (UL). There are neither adverse effects nor documented benefits associated with exceeding the recommended intake, provided intake remains below the UL. Planning is always for *usual* intake, defined as an individual's intake over a long period of time.

In some cases it may be appropriate to use a target other than the RDA for individuals. The RDA provides assurance that the probability of inadequacy does not exceed 2 to 3 percent. However, nutritionists and other planners may decide to use a different definition of what is an acceptably low probability of nutrient inadequacy. If so, the rationale should be clearly stated.

The EAR is *not* used as a goal in planning individual diets. By definition, a diet planned to provide the EAR of a nutrient would have a 50 percent probability of not meeting an individual's requirement, and this is an unacceptable degree of risk for the individual.

The situation for energy is quite different. In this case, there are adverse effects to individuals who consume intake above their requirements—over time, weight gain will occur. This difference is reflected in the fact that there is no RDA for energy, as it would be inappropriate to recommend an intake that exceeded the requirement of 97 to 98 percent of individuals. The only DRI available for energy is the EER (estimated energy requirement), which reflects the estimated average energy expenditure associated with an individual's sex, age, height, weight, and physical activity level. As such, it exceeds the needs of half the individuals with specified characteristics, and is below the needs of the other half. Although the EER may be used as an initial planning goal, body weight must be monitored and intake adjusted as appropriate.

Finally, it is necessary to consider the recommended distribution of energy from the macronutrients fat, carbohydrate, and protein (IOM, 2002a). For example, for adults, their energy consumed from fat should be between 20 and 35 percent.

Developing Dietary Plans

Dietary plans will usually be developed using food-based dietary guidance. In the past, dietary reference standards (e.g., the former RDAs in the United States and Recommended Nutrient Intakes in Canada) have been used to provide food-based dietary guidance in several ways. These include developing national food guides and dietary guidelines for healthy individuals, providing consumer information on food and supplement labels, and serving as a reference standard for nutrient content and health claims. When dietary reference standards are revised, there will be unavoidable time lags until food guides and information on food and supplement labels are assessed and revised, if necessary, to reflect the new nutrient standards. When these gaps occur, diets of individuals must be planned using more detailed data on nutrient composition, such as those found in food composition databases. Information on food and supplement labels may be useful for estimating macronutrient contents (e.g., energy, fat, and fiber), but may be less useful in situations where the labeling reference standards do not reflect the current recommended intakes. Planners may wish to start with current food guides and then check to be certain that the resulting diets meet the RDAs and AIs without exceeding the ULs.

The Bottom Line: Planning Individual Diets

The goal of planning diets for individuals is to have a low probability of inadequacy while minimizing potential risk of excess for each nutrient. In most cases, this is done by meeting the RDA or AI while not exceeding the UL. This can be accomplished by using food guides such as *Canada's Food Guide to Healthy Eating* (Health Canada, 1991) or the U.S. Food Guide Pyramid (USDA, 1992), although supplemental information such as food composition databases should also be used in situations when these guides may not reflect the DRIs. Gaps or excesses identified can then be remedied by planning to alter the type or amount of foods in the various food groups, by using fortified foods, or by using supplements.

USING DIETARY REFERENCE INTAKES TO PLAN DIETS FOR GROUPS

Planning diets for groups is a multistep process. It involves identifying the specific nutritional goals, determining how best to achieve these goals, and, ultimately, assessing if these goals are achieved.

The goal of planning for groups is to determine a distribution of usual nutrient intakes that provides for a low prevalence of inadequate intakes and a low prevalence of intakes that may be at potential risk of adverse effects due to excessive intake. This proposed framework thus shifts the focus of planning away from using dietary recommendations in deciding what to offer or serve to what is ultimately desired in terms of the distribution of usual nutrient intakes in the group.

By focusing explicitly on the distribution of usual nutrient intakes of a group, the framework for planning presented below is, in many respects, a new paradigm.

The procedures used for planning intakes of groups differ depending on whether the group is relatively homogeneous (e.g., a single life stage and gender group, such as women 31 to 50 years of age), or is composed of a number of subgroups that differ in nutrient and energy requirements.

Planning for Homogeneous Groups

The important steps in planning diets for a homogeneous group include:

• selecting the goals, including the acceptable prevalence of inadequacy and prevalence of intakes at risk of excessive intake, for each nutrient of interest;
• estimating the target usual intake distributions for each nutrient;
• planning a menu to achieve the target usual intake distributions; and
• assessing the results of the planning.

Selecting the Goals

The first step in planning for groups is to select the goals: what will be considered an acceptable prevalence of inadequate intakes and what will be considered an acceptable prevalence of intakes at potential risk of adverse effects. These decisions need to be made for each nutrient of interest that has an Estimated Average Requirement (EAR) or Tolerable Upper Intake Level (UL). One approach is to aim for a prevalence of inadequacy of 2 to 3 percent and a prevalence of intakes at risk of adverse effects of 2 to 3 percent.

However, higher or lower prevalences could be selected for either, and the selected prevalences may vary by nutrient.

Goals may also be set for nutrients with an Adequate Intake (AI). In these cases, the goal will usually be to achieve a median intake equal to the AI. For energy intake, the goal is to provide the mean estimated energy requirement (EER) for the group. In addition, planners will usually wish to specify goals related to macronutrient distribution, such as ensuring that the energy from fat is between 20 and 35 percent for adults.

Estimating the Target Usual Nutrient Intake Distribution

For nutrients with an EAR, the next step in planning group diets is to determine the usual intake distribution that will meet these goals. This process needs to be repeated for each nutrient of interest.

A target usual nutrient intake distribution has an acceptably low prevalence of inadequate or excessive intakes, as defined by the proportion of individuals in the group with usual intakes less than requirements or greater than the UL. In most cases, the prevalence of inadequate intakes is estimated as the proportion of the group below the EAR, and the prevalence of excessive intakes is estimated as the proportion of the group above the UL.

In order to select a target usual nutrient intake distribution, it is necessary to make some assumptions about usual intake distributions for the group of interest. In some cases, the planner may have information on the current intake distribution for the group, and can use this information to plan the new intake distribution. In other cases, it will be necessary to use intake distributions from similar groups (for example, using data from national nutrition surveys). In either case, the distribution of *usual* intakes is needed, with the effect of day-to-day variation removed. Because intake distributions are seldom normal, it is usually not possible to determine the distribution from just the mean and standard deviation of intakes. Percentiles of intakes are almost always needed.

Next, the planner needs to position the intake distribution so the nutrient intake goals are met. For example, if a planner decides that the prevalence of inadequacy in the group should be set at 2 to 3 percent, then the usual nutrient intake distribution of the group should be positioned such that only 2 to 3 percent of individuals in the group have usual intake less than the EAR. Using the EAR as a cut-point for estimating the prevalence of inadequate intakes builds directly on the approaches previously described for assessing intakes (IOM, 2000a).

It is appropriate to use the EAR as a cut-point for estimating the prevalence of inadequate intakes for all nutrients with an EAR, except iron. Because the iron requirements are not normally distributed, it is necessary to use published tables showing the distribution of iron requirements in order to estimate the prevalence of inadequate intakes (IOM, 2001).

Because the available intake distribution will not usually be correctly positioned to meet the nutrient goals, the planner must move it up (or down) by adding (or subtracting) a constant amount of the nutrient to each point on the distribution until the appropriate prevalences are obtained. When the distribution is correctly positioned, it becomes the target usual intake distribution.

Assuming there are no changes in the shape of the distribution, the amount of the shift can be calculated as the additional amount of the nutrient that must be consumed to reduce the proportion of the group that is below the EAR. For example, the EAR for zinc for girls 9 to 13 years old is 7 mg/day. Current data from the Third National Health and Nutrition Examination Survey show that about 10 percent of the girls have intakes below the EAR. If the goal is to plan intakes so that only 2 to 3 percent are below the EAR, intakes need to be increased. The amount of the increase can be calculated as the difference between the current intake at the 2nd to 3rd percentile (which is 6.2 mg/day) and the desired intake at the 2nd to 3rd percentile (the EAR of 7 mg/day); the difference is thus 0.8 mg/day. That means that the distribution of intakes needs to shift up by 0.8 mg/day in order to have only 2 to 3 percent of the girls with intakes below the EAR.

The same procedure should be followed to determine if the distribution meets the goal of a low prevalence of potentially excessive intakes. For zinc, the UL for girls 9 to 13 years of age is 23 mg/day. The 99th percentile of their current usual intake distribution is 15.5 mg/day, so even if the distribution is shifted up by 0.8 mg/day, the 99th percentile (16.3 mg/day) is below the UL.

The median of the target intake distribution is a useful summary measure, as it can be used as an initial tool in planning menus. Assuming that the shape of the intake distribution does not change as a result of planning, the median of the target intake distribution is calculated as the median of the current usual intake distribution, plus (or minus) the amount that the distribution needs to shift to make it the target usual nutrient intake distribution. In the zinc example above, the distribution needed to shift by an additional 0.8 mg/day. The median of the current zinc distribution for these girls is 9.4 mg/day, so the median of the target usual intake distribution would be 9.4 + 0.8 = 10.2 mg/day.

The median of a target intake distribution will usually exceed the Recommended Dietary Allowance (RDA) because the variance in usual intakes exceeds the variance in requirements. The RDA for zinc for girls is 8 mg/day, but the target median intake is 10.2 mg/day. Thus, selection of the RDA as the median of the target usual intake distribution is not recommended as it results in a percentage of inadequacy greater than would likely be selected with more careful consideration.

Planning a Menu to Achieve the Target Usual Intake Distributions

After the planner has estimated a target usual intake distribution for each nutrient of interest, this information needs to be operationalized into a menu. Menu planning involves several steps:

1. Establishing an initial goal for the nutrient content of the menu that is based on the target usual nutrient intake distribution.
2. Determining what foods to offer that will most likely result in a distribution of usual nutrient intake that approximates the target, and thus attains the desired prevalence of nutrient adequacy.
3. Determining the quantities of foods to purchase and serve.

Step 1. Establish an initial goal for the nutrient content of the menu.

It might appear logical to use the median of the target usual intake distribution as a goal for the nutrient content of a menu. As described earlier, this would be projected to lead to an intake distribution with the desired prevalence of nutrient adequacy, assuming that the shape of the distribution did not change. However, in almost all group-feeding situations, nutrient *intakes* are less than the nutrient content of the foods *provided* (i.e., food is not completely consumed). Furthermore, many planning applications involve offering a variety of menu options from which the members of the group will select foods. For these reasons, the planner might aim for a menu that offers a variety of meals with a nutrient content range that includes, or even exceeds, the median of the target nutrient intake distribution.

It is necessary to set initial planning goals for all nutrients of interest. For nutrients with an AI, it is not possible to estimate the prevalence of inadequacy, and the goal should be to achieve median intakes at the AI. Thus, the AI can be used as a planning goal if the distribution of intakes for the group of interest is similar to the distribution of intakes that was used when setting the AI. For energy intake, either a mean EER or the mean of the current energy intake distribution should be determined. An EER may be calculated for a reference person that is typical for the group of interest, or more accurately, by using an average EER for the members of the group. However, accurate estimates of heights, weights, and physical activity levels are needed to estimate an energy requirement, and these are often not available. Thus, even though it is known that energy intakes are often underreported, the mean of the distribution of energy intakes may also be used as the target in the planning process. In either case, monitoring of body weight should occur.

Step 2. Determine what foods to offer.

After all the nutrient targets have been set, the planner must select foods that will provide this average level of nutrient intake. To convert nutrient intake targets into food intakes, planners will usually rely on food guides such as the U.S. Food Guide Pyramid (USDA, 1992), *Canada's Food Guide to Healthy Eating* (Health Canada, 1991), published menus, and previously used menus to design a menu that is likely to result in the target level of adequacy. This will typically be an iterative process, often assisted by nutrient calculation software that allows interactive changes to menus and then recalculates the nutrient levels at each step. In addition to achieving goals for prevalence of inadequate intakes and prevalence of potentially excessive intakes, goals for acceptable macronutrient distribution ranges (IOM, 2002a) will also need to be considered.

Step 3. Determine the quantities of foods to purchase, offer, and serve.

Designing menu *offerings* to meet an *intake* target is a difficult task. Because food selections and plate waste vary among groups, and among menus within groups, the appropriate procedures for determining the foods to offer depend heavily on the particular planning context. In addition, the amount to purchase to be able to offer or serve must take into account food waste due to preparation losses.

Assessing the Results of the Plan

The final step in planning intakes is to assess the results of the planning process. Such an assessment would follow the procedures for assessing group intakes (IOM, 2000a). There are several reasons why assessment is a crucial component of the framework for group planning.

First, planners typically can control only what is offered to individuals in the group, not what they actually eat. Because the goal of planning is to achieve an acceptable group prevalence of inadequate nutrient intakes, it is clear that to judge the success of the planning activity, assessment of intakes must occur.

Furthermore, the distribution of intakes that was chosen as the starting point for the planning activity often will not be taken from the group whose intakes are being planned. For example, it may be necessary to start with intake distributions from national surveys. Thus, the planner is making an assumption about the applicability of the distribution to the group of interest.

In addition, a crucial assumption was made when selecting the target median intake—that shifting the distribution of intakes to a new position would not change the shape of the distribution. If the shape changes, then the estimated target median intake may be incorrect. The shape of the distribution is likely to depend on many factors, including food preferences, the types of foods served, and the amount of food needed to meet each person's energy needs. Thus, there are several reasons to believe the distribution's shape may change if a different selection of foods were served. This is another reason why assessment is a crucial component of good planning.

Planning group diets is an iterative, ongoing effort in which planners set goals for usual intake, plan menus to achieve these goals, provide these new menus, assess whether the planning was successful, and then modify their planning procedures accordingly.

Planning for Nonhomogeneous Groups

If nutrient or energy requirements (or both) are not uniform across a group, the approach to planning can vary. In some cases it may be possible to target the most vulnerable subgroup (i.e., that with the highest nutrient requirements relative to energy needs) for a specific intervention. In other cases it may not be possible or practical to target the vulnerable subgroup, and in these situations, a nutrient density approach can be used. Even within a group with the same nutrient requirements, energy requirements may vary substantially, and the nutrient density approach may also be applicable.

Nutrient density is defined as the ratio of the content of a nutrient to the energy provided by the food item, diet, or food supply. It is expressed as the unit weight of the nutrient per 1,000 kcal or per MJ of energy.

A simple nutrient density approach for heterogeneous groups is to determine the subgroup with the highest target median nutrient intake *relative to their estimated average energy requirement.* Energy requirements can be obtained by using the current average energy intake of the subgroup, or by calculating the average EER for the subgroup. For example, in a hypothetical group of men and women combined, assume that the vitamin C target median intake for the men is 138 mg/day, and the target median intake for the women is 116 mg/day. If the average EER for the men is 2,600 kcal/day, then their target median vitamin C intake, expressed as a density, is 138/2.6, or 52 mg/1,000 kcal. If the average EER for the women is 1,800 kcal/day, then their target median intake, expressed as a density, is 116/1.8, or 64 mg/1,000 kcal. Thus, the women require a higher vitamin C density in their diets. In this simple approach, the planner would use the target median vitamin C density for the women in the menu planning process, and would assume that the men's intake would also be adequate.

However, the simple approach does not consider the actual distribution of nutrient densities within the group. A new method of planning for heterogeneous groups is proposed in this report. Its goal is to develop a *target nutrient density distribution* for each subgroup, and then choose the highest target median density from these distributions as the nutrient density to be used in planning. There are three steps to deriving a target usual nutrient density intake distribution:

1. Obtain the target distribution of usual nutrient intakes for each subgroup of interest.
2. Combine the target distribution of usual nutrient intakes with the usual energy intake distribution in each subgroup to obtain the target distribution of usual nutrient intakes expressed as densities.
3. Compare the estimated target median intake density for each discrete subgroup to identify the highest nutrient density and use this density to set planning targets for the whole group.

This approach is theoretically more likely to provide an accurate estimate of the appropriate target median intakes for heterogeneous groups, although the practicality of its use in planning has not been tested.

For either the simple approach or the target nutrient density distribution approach, this selection process would then be repeated for each nutrient of interest for the group, and planning a menu to achieve these targets would proceed as described above.

For some nutrients (notably iron), prioritization of the needs of the subgroup with the highest requirement relative to energy can result in the selection of a target median intake that far exceeds the needs of all other subgroups. Under these circumstances, planners must consider the risk that members of subgroups with lower nutrient requirements relative to energy may achieve intake levels in excess of the UL. In such situations, it may be preferable to target the vulnerable subgroups through education or supplementation.

Because the simple approach does not consider the distribution of nutrient densities, and the target nutrient density distribution approach is currently untested, it is particularly important to assess nutrient intakes as a final step in the process of planning for groups.

SPECIAL CONSIDERATIONS

When using the Dietary Reference Intakes (DRIs) for planning dietary intakes, it is helpful to consider the process and criteria used for developing the DRIs for specific nutrients. Special considerations for planning include factors that affect nutrient bioavailability, such as the source, chemical form, and dietary matrix, as well as the physiological, lifestyle, and health factors that may alter nutrient requirements and therefore recommended intakes. These factors need to be considered whether planning diets for individuals or for groups.

Both planning and assessment often rely on self-reported intake, and thus it is important to consider the well-documented issue of underreporting of energy intakes and its effects on the accuracy of self-reported *nutrient* intakes. If intakes are underreported, then the planner may start the planning process with incorrect data on current intakes and may also incorrectly assess the results of the planning process. Unfortunately, well-accepted, validated methods to statistically correct for the effects of underreporting the estimated distribution of usual intakes are presently lacking. If planners have the means to measure intakes (e.g., by observing foods selected and food wasted by patients in a nursing home), the results of the planning and subsequent assessment will be more valid than self-reported intakes for almost all groups.

RESEARCH IMPLICATIONS AND RECOMMENDATIONS

Several crucial areas have been identified where data and techniques do not exist or additional knowledge is needed. These needs are synthesized and prioritized in several key areas, including research on dietary planning for groups, improving the quality of dietary intake data, providing guidance for dietary planning, and improving estimates of nutrient requirements. These areas are summarized below.

Implementing Dietary Planning for Groups

• Pilot test the approaches to dietary planning for groups that are proposed in this report. The approach to group planning proposed in this report is a new paradigm, and should be tested in pilot studies before being implemented on a larger scale.

• Determine how different nutrition interventions affect intake distributions. Examination and publication of intake distributions before and after an intervention, with a systematic collection of this type of data, would allow a more informed selection of methods for planning a dietary intervention.

• Determine the intake distributions of specific population groups. Although data on dietary intakes may be available either from national population surveys or surveys of large groups, often such information has not been reported in a manner that facilitates the estimation of variations in the usual intake of individuals.

• Determine the relationship between foods offered and nutrient intake in the context of group planning. Research is needed to determine how food offerings relate to food and nutrient intakes, and how the relationship between food offered and intake varies according to planning context.

• Develop and evaluate dietary planning strategies for heterogeneous groups, including a nutrient density approach to dietary planning. Research is needed to determine the practical usefulness of planning for a target nutrient density, determine if the applicability of the nutrient density approach is limited to situations with predetermined food allocations or restricted food choices (e.g., emergency relief rations), and determine if this approach would be practical in situations offering a wide variety of food choices, where the nutrient density is more dependent on food selection than on total food access to meet energy needs.

Improving the Quality of Dietary Intake Data

Much has been written about ways to improve the quality of the intake data on which dietary assessment and planning are based; a number of these issues were discussed in a previous report (IOM, 2000a) and are reiterated here.

- Develop and validate statistical procedures to identify and correct for both under- and overreporting in self-reported intake data for energy and other nutrients.
- Identify and validate better ways to quantify the intake of supplements.
- Update food composition databases to include the forms and units that are specified by the DRIs.

Developing Approaches to Providing Guidance for Dietary Planning

- Review and, where necessary, revise existing food guides.
- Develop technical tools for the professional.
- Educate nutrition professionals about correct uses of the DRIs.
- Assess application of the DRIs for food and supplement labeling.
- Develop and evaluate food guides for group planning.

Improving Estimates of Nutrient Requirements

- Improve existing estimates of the Estimated Average Requirement (EAR) and Recommended Dietary Allowance.
- Provide better information on requirements so it becomes possible to establish an EAR for nutrients that currently have Adequate Intakes.
- Improve estimates of the distribution of requirements so that the appropriate method for assessing the prevalence of inadequacy for groups can be determined (cut-point method versus probability approach).
- Identify the factors that can alter the upper intake levels that can be tolerated biologically.

1

Introduction to Dietary Planning

This report is one of a series of publications resulting from a comprehensive effort initiated by the Institute of Medicine's Food and Nutrition Board in 1993 to expand the approach to the development of dietary reference standards. The new categories of reference values have specific uses and thus are a significant departure from the previous Recommended Dietary Allowances (RDAs) in the United States and Recommended Nutrient Intakes (RNIs) in Canada. The focus of this report is to examine the appropriate use of each of the available types of Dietary Reference Intake (DRI) values in planning nutrient intakes of groups and individuals.

This report should be of particular use to nutrition and public health researchers in their work, to dietitians and nutritionists responsible for the education of the next generation of practitioners, and to the government professionals involved in the development and implementation of national diet and health assessments, public education efforts, and food assistance programs. The report reviews the statistical underpinnings for the application of the various types of DRI values in planning, illustrates sample applications, and provides guidelines to help professionals determine when specific uses are appropriate or inappropriate.

Planners need to have a good understanding of the DRIs, including how each requirement was derived, and whether the Tolerable Upper Intake Levels were based on all sources of nutrients or just fortificants and supplements. An understanding of basic statistics is also needed, especially for group planners. Planners must understand the concepts of risk and probability.

BACKGROUND

The term *Dietary Reference Intakes* (DRIs) refers to a set of nutrient-based reference values, each of which has special uses. The development of DRIs expands on the periodic reports called *Recommended Dietary Allowances* (RDAs), which have been published since 1941 by the U.S. National Academies, and the Canadian Dietary Standards, called *Recommended Nutrient Intakes* (RNIs) published since 1938 by the Canadian government. This comprehensive effort has been undertaken by the Standing Committee on the Scientific Evaluation of Dietary Reference Intakes of the Food and Nutrition Board, Institute of Medicine, National Academies, at the request of the U.S. government and Health Canada.

A previous report in this series (IOM, 2000a) examined the use of DRIs in dietary assessment for individuals and groups. Dietary assessment, whether for an individual or a group, compares usual nutrient intakes with estimated nutrient requirements and examines the probability of inadequate or excessive intake. Dietary planning, on the other hand, aims for the consumption of diets that have acceptably low probabilities of inadequate or excessive nutrient intakes.

Dietary planning involves using the DRIs to set goals for what intakes should be.

Dietary planning may be done at several different levels. It may refer to an individual planning a meal and making relevant food purchases, a food service manager in an institution planning daily menus, or a government agency planning large nutrition or food assistance programs. For the purposes of this report, dietary planning applies to planning intake, rather than the amount of food purchased or served.

Nutritional considerations are only one component of dietary planning. Other considerations include incorporating food preferences of the individual or group being planned for, and the cost and availability of foods. However, using estimates of nutrient requirements to set intake goals should be part of the planning activity.

Figure 1-1 illustrates a conceptual framework described by Beaton (1994) that can be applied to the interpretation and uses of the DRIs. As shown in the framework, knowledge about both nutrient requirements and nutrient intakes feeds into two general applications: diet planning and diet assessment. Within each of these general categories, the applications differ according to whether they are for an individual or for population groups.

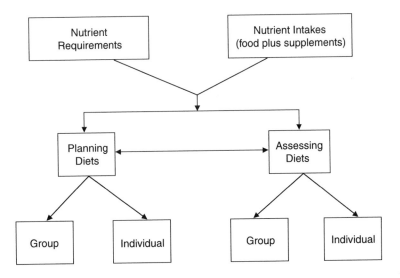

FIGURE 1-1 Conceptual framework—uses of dietary reference standards.
SOURCE: Adapted from Beaton (1994).

The simplicity of the above statements belies the complexity in using and interpreting DRIs to plan and assess diets. Two important factors account for this complexity. In the past, both planning and assessment applications have relied primarily on the former RDAs and RNIs because these were the only nutrient standards widely available. Often, the concepts underlying the former RDAs and RNIs were not well understood, and thus some applications for both assessment and planning purposes were inappropriate (IOM, 1994). Therefore, additional types of reference intakes have been developed (Estimated Average Requirement, Adequate Intake, and Tolerable Upper Intake Level). With the three additional categories of dietary reference intakes now available, applications need to be carefully considered and clearly explained so each of the categories are used appropriately. DRIs can be used in situations such as planning individual diets; planning nutrition and food procurement for the military, prisons, nursing homes, and other institutionalized groups; food labeling and nutritional marketing; clinical dietetics; food fortification; developing new or modified food products; and assessing food safety.

The approaches discussed in this report for using the DRIs as a guide in planning dietary intakes for individuals and for groups rely on the same basic principles that were presented in the previous report on applications of the DRIs in dietary assessment (IOM, 2000a). Those principles provide the rationale for using each of the DRIs for individual and group diet assessment, and the same rationale extends to the use of the DRIs in diet planning.

WHAT ARE DIETARY REFERENCE INTAKES?

As indicated above, the term *Dietary Reference Intakes* (DRIs) refers to a set of at least four nutrient-based reference values that can be used for planning and assessing diets and for many other purposes. An important principle underlying both the former Recommended Dietary Allowances (RDAs) and Recommended Nutrition Intakes (RNIs) and the new DRIs is that *these are standards for healthy people— they are not appropriate for individuals or groups who are ill or for repletion of deficient individuals.*

The concepts underlying the new DRIs differ from the former RDAs and RNIs as indicated in Box 1-1.

Processes Used to Establish the Dietary Reference Intakes

In establishing the EAR or Adequate Intake (AI) for nutrients, a requirement is defined as the lowest continuing intake level of a

---

BOX 1-1 New Concepts Underlying the DRIs

• Where specific data on safety and a role in health exist, reduction in the risk of chronic degenerative disease or developmental abnormality, rather than just the absence of signs of deficiency, is included in the formulation of the recommendation.

• The concepts of probability and risk explicitly underpin the determination of the Estimated Average Requirement (EAR), RDA, and Tolerable Upper Intake Level (UL) and inform their application in assessment and planning.

• ULs are established where data exist regarding risk of adverse health effects.

• Compounds found naturally in food that may not meet the traditional concept of a nutrient but have potential risk or possible benefit to health are reviewed, and if sufficient data exist, reference intakes are established.

nutrient that will maintain a defined level of nutriture in an individual. The chosen criterion of nutritional adequacy upon which this requirement is based is different for each nutrient and is identified in the DRI nutrient reports (IOM, 1997, 1998a, 2000b, 2001, 2002a). In some cases, the criteria may differ for individuals at different life stages for the same nutrient. In developing the DRIs, emphasis is placed on the reasons underlying the particular criterion of adequacy used to establish the requirement for each nutrient. A more detailed discussion of the origin and framework of the DRIs is presented in Appendix A.

The EARs are based on a thorough review of the scientific literature for health outcomes associated with the nutrient. The criteria and evidence-based rationale used for setting each EAR are clearly specified. An estimate of the variation in the requirement is also specified, and is used to set the RDA. When data are inadequate to establish an EAR and RDA, other approaches are used to establish an intake goal, which is designated an AI. The process used to establish the UL involves the estimation of an uncertainty factor that is applied to a no-observed-adverse-effect level (NOAEL) or to a lowest-observed-adverse-effect level (LOAEL) based on human or animal data related to identified hazards.

Estimated Average Requirement[1]

The *Estimated Average Requirement* (EAR) is the usual intake level that is estimated to meet the requirement of half the healthy individuals in a life stage and gender group. At this level of intake, the other half of the healthy individuals in the specified group would not have their needs met. The EAR is based on a specific criterion of adequacy, derived from a careful review of the literature. When selecting the criterion, reduction of disease risk is considered along with many other health parameters. For example, the EAR for vitamin C is based on "an amount thought to provide antioxidant protection as derived from the correlation of such protection with neutrophil ascorbate concentrations" (IOM, 2000b). For energy,

---

[1] It is recognized that the definition of EAR implies a median as opposed to a mean or average. The median and average would be the same if the distribution of requirements followed a symmetric distribution, and would diverge as the distribution became skewed. Two considerations prompted the choice of the term EAR: (1) data are rarely adequate to determine the distribution of requirements, and (2) precedent has been set by other countries that have used the term EAR for reference values similarly derived (COMA, 1991).

the situation is somewhat different. Energy requirements are estimated on an individual basis using a person's gender, age, height, weight, and physical activity level to estimate total energy expenditure; thus the specific criterion of adequacy is maintenance of a healthy body mass index with a healthy level of physical activity.

Recommended Dietary Allowance

The *Recommended Dietary Allowance* (RDA) is the dietary intake level that is sufficient to meet the nutrient requirement of nearly all healthy individuals in a particular life stage and gender group. If the distribution of requirements in the group is assumed to be normal, the RDA is computed from the EAR by adding two standard deviations of the requirement (SD_{REQ}) as follows:

$$RDA = EAR + 2\ SD_{REQ}$$

The standard deviation of the requirement distribution can be observed directly if sufficient data are available. Often this is not the case, and the standard deviation is estimated by assuming a specific coefficient of variation (CV) for the average requirement. A CV of 10 percent has been used for many nutrients (IOM, 1997, 1998a, 2000b, 2001), and for these, the RDA equals 120 percent of the EAR. Therefore, assuming a normal distribution, 97 to 98 percent of the individuals in the group will have a requirement that is below the RDA. If the distribution of requirements is known to be skewed rather than normal (for example, iron requirements of menstruating women), the RDA is obtained by finding the usual intake level that is at the 97th to 98th percentile of the requirement distribution. In either case, the RDA developed in the DRI process differs conceptually from the former RDAs and RNIs since with the establishment of an EAR, the RDA is determined quantitatively rather than through the use of judgment-based safety factors.

The RDA is intended for use primarily as a goal for intake of individuals. Because the RDA is often derived directly from the EAR and an estimate of variability of the requirement distribution, if data are insufficient to establish an EAR, no RDA can be set.

Adequate Intake

If sufficient scientific evidence is not available to establish an EAR, and thus determine an RDA, a reference intake called an *Adequate Intake* (AI) may be derived instead. The AI is a value based on experimentally derived levels of intake or the mean nutrient intake by a group (or groups) of apparently healthy people who are maintaining a defined nutritional state or criterion of adequacy. Examples of defined nutritional states include normal growth, maintenance of normal circulating nutrient values or biochemical indices, or other characteristics of nutritional well-being or general health related to the nutrient.

For example, the AI for young infants is based on the daily mean nutrient intake supplied by human milk for healthy, full-term infants who are exclusively breastfed. For adults, the AI may be based on data from a single experiment (e.g., the AI for choline [IOM, 1998a]), on estimated dietary intakes in apparently healthy population groups (e.g., the AI for pantothenic acid [IOM, 1998a]), or on combined data from different approaches (e.g., usual dietary intake and experimentally altered intakes of calcium in adult women [IOM, 1997]). The AI is thus expected to exceed the true EAR (and often the RDA) if it could be set for the same specified criterion of nutritional adequacy. In the absence of an EAR (and RDA) for a nutrient, the AI can be used as the intake goal.

The issuance of an AI is an indication that more research is needed to determine with confidence the mean and distribution of requirements for a specific nutrient. As this research is completed, it should be possible to replace estimates of AIs with EARs and RDAs.

Tolerable Upper Intake Level

The *Tolerable Upper Intake Level* (UL) is the highest level of continuing daily nutrient intake that is likely to pose no risk of adverse health effects to almost all individuals in a specified life stage and gender group. As intake increases above the UL, the potential risk of adverse health effects increases. The term *tolerable intake* was chosen to avoid implying a possible beneficial effect from levels of intakes above the RDA. Instead, the term is intended to connote a level of intake that can, with high probability, be tolerated biologically. The UL is not a recommended level of intake, and there is no currently established benefit to healthy individuals associated with ingestion of nutrients in amounts exceeding the RDA or AI.

The UL is based on an evaluation conducted using the methodology for risk assessment of the adverse effects of nutrients (IOM, 1999). (A detailed explanation of this methodology is also included in all of the DRI nutrient reports.) The need to establish ULs grew in part out of the increased fortification of foods with nutrients and the increased use of dietary supplements. Details are given for each nutrient on how the UL was established (IOM, 1997, 1998a, 2000b, 2001, 2002a). For some nutrients there may be insufficient data on which to develop a UL. The lack of a UL cannot be interpreted as meaning that high intake poses no risk of adverse effects.

Unless otherwise stated in the DRI nutrient reports, values given for EARs, RDAs, AIs, and ULs are based on the total intake of the nutrient naturally occurring in food, added to food as a fortificant, and from supplements.

IMPLEMENTATION OF DIETARY PLANNING FOR INDIVIDUALS AND GROUPS

Planning diets refers to determining what usual nutrient intake should be. Regardless of whether one is planning diets for individuals or groups, the goal is to have diets that are nutritionally adequate, or conversely, to ensure that the probability of nutrient inadequacy or excess is acceptably low. As will be described in depth in this report, how this goal is implemented differs when planning for individuals compared to planning for groups. Nevertheless, the underlying considerations are similar.

At the individual level, usual intake is defined as the individual's average intake over a long period of time. As discussed in greater detail in the Dietary Reference Intake (DRI) report on dietary assessment (IOM, 2000a), because of the large day-to-day variation in individual intake, intake on one or even several days may provide inaccurate estimates of an individual's usual intake. Similarly, for groups, the focus for diet planning is the distribution of usual intake, which is the distribution of the long-term average intakes of individuals in the group. Usual intake distributions can be estimated by adjusting the observed intake distributions using statistical techniques (NRC, 1986; Nusser et al., 1996). By removing the day-to-day variation in intakes (within-person variation), the resulting adjusted distribution better reflects the individual-to-individual variation of intakes within the group.

Another consideration in the implementation of dietary planning is the concept of an acceptably low probability of nutrient inadequacy (probability that intake does not meet requirement) or, conversely, a high probability of nutrient adequacy. For individuals, an acceptably low probability of nutrient inadequacy has been traditionally accomplished by planning for the individual's usual intake to be at the Recommended Dietary Allowance for the nutrient, such that the probability of inadequacy does not exceed 2 to 3 percent.

To date, planning for groups has generally not incorporated planning for a low prevalence of nutrient inadequacy, in large part because the tools required (knowledge of the Estimated Average Requirement and the usual intake distribution) have not been widely available. Thus, there is no convention about what prevalence of inadequacy is acceptably low. It is in the professional judgment of the nutritionist or planner to determine what is an acceptably low probability of nutrient inadequacy for an individual or prevalence of inadequacy for groups. The level selected should be clearly stated. Similarly, in applying the DRIs for planning, professional judgment is required to determine the likelihood of any recognized benefit of increasing intakes beyond their current level.

CAVEATS REGARDING THE USE OF DIETARY REFERENCE INTAKES IN DIETARY PLANNING AND ASSESSMENT

Dietary planning and assessment are inextricably linked. Assessment is used as a basis for planning and to evaluate whether the planning goals have been met. Those assessing and planning diets should be aware of limitations in the data that underpin the Dietary Reference Intakes (DRIs) and their application: there is uncertainty associated with the estimates of the Estimated Average Requirements (EARs) themselves, and dietary intake and food composition data are subject to inaccuracy.

Limitations in the Data on Nutrient Requirements

Detailed consideration of the DRI reports for specific nutrients (IOM, 1997, 1998a, 2000b, 2001, 2002a) can provide insight into both what is known and what information is still needed to further define intakes that support health. In interpreting the DRIs for use in dietary planning, planners should be aware that often the EARs are based on data from a limited number of individuals; that for most nutrients the precise variation in requirements is not known and has been approximated from the variation in related physiological parameters; that, in the absence of evidence to the contrary, the variation in individual requirements has been assumed to follow a normal distribution; that the EAR has often been extrapolated from one population group to others that differ in life stage and gender; and that the degree of uncertainty associated with the EAR has not been specified. By definition, EARs are estimates—they are not defined with 100 percent accuracy. Thus, although the best available evidence was used, gaps in the knowledge base remain.

Choice of Requirement Criterion

Knowledge of the criterion used by the DRI panels to determine the EAR and Recommended Dietary Allowance (RDA) can help in assessing the potential impact of not meeting these guidelines. This may affect setting goals for nutrient intake, including selection of an acceptable group prevalence of dietary inadequacy (e.g., the proportion of a group with intakes below the EAR).

In establishing the DRIs, the requirements for most nutrients have been presented as a single endpoint for various life stage and gender groups, rather than as multiple endpoints. To the extent that for most nutrients a single endpoint has been established for an EAR and RDA, this approach differs from that originally recommended by NRC (1986) and adopted by the Joint Food and Agriculture Organization and World Health Organization Expert Consultation on the requirements of vitamin A, iron, folate, and B_{12} (FAO/WHO, 1988). These groups recommended both a basal requirement level (the amount of nutrient needed to prevent a clinically detectable impairment of function) and a normative storage requirement level (the amount of nutrient needed to maintain a desirable level in tissues). However, the DRI process does allow for multiple endpoints to be used where the data exist, and to date this has been done for vitamin A. An EAR has been set for the reversal of night blindness, and an EAR and RDA have also been set for the maintenance of liver stores. A planner might want to ensure that intakes would result in a minimal (near zero) prevalence of inadequacy with regard to night blindness, but might be willing to accept, and thus plan for, a somewhat higher prevalence of inadequacy with regard to maintenance of normal liver stores.

Inadequate Dietary Intake Versus Inadequate Nutritional Status

Planning diets for groups involves choosing an acceptable group prevalence of dietary inadequacy (see Chapter 3). Theoretically, this would correspond to the prevalence of inadequate nutritional status with regard to the criterion used to establish the EAR. For example, if planners chose to maintain the current distribution of vitamin B_6 intake in the United States in women aged 31 to 50 (see appendixes to the DRI publications for tables describing the population distributions of nutrient intakes [IOM 1997, 1998a, 2000b, 2001, 2002]), they would be accepting an apparent group prevalence of dietary inadequacy between 10 and 15 percent, according to data from the Third National Health and Nutrition Examination

Survey (NHANES III). If the assumptions involved in establishing the EAR were correct and applied to all population groups, one would expect to observe similar proportions consuming vitamin B_6 below the EAR and with low plasma pyridoxal phosphate levels (i.e., inadequate nutritional status with regard to the indicator used to set the EAR). In practice, however, the apparent prevalence of *dietary inadequacy* of a nutrient may not be equivalent to the prevalence of *inadequate nutritional status* for the same nutrient.

Sources of error contributing to any observed discrepancies between estimates of the prevalence of inadequate intake and inadequate nutritional status include those involved in estimating dietary intakes. These have been reviewed in the DRI report on dietary assessment (IOM, 2000a), and include an incomplete knowledge of (1) the nutrient composition of foods, (2) the nutrient bioavailability from different food and supplemental sources, (3) the usual intakes as compared with short-term intakes, and (4) the under-reporting of self-reported dietary intakes. The uncertainties involved in estimating nutrient requirements can also contribute to observed discrepancies, as can the lack of population data on the biochemical indicators of nutrient adequacy used to establish the requirement estimates.

Sources of Error in Planning for Dietary Intake

Uncertainty of Requirement Estimates

For some nutrients, the sources of error in estimating intakes and requirements are not extreme, and the apparent prevalence of dietary inadequacy (e.g., the proportion below the EAR) corresponds reasonably well to the prevalence of inadequate nutritional status with regard to the criterion used to establish the EAR. For example, the EAR for iron was established as the amount of iron needed to meet body functions with minimal storage, and this was determined to be reflected by a serum ferritin concentration of about 15 µg/L (IOM, 2001). When the prevalence of inadequate iron intakes was compared to the prevalence of apparent biochemical deficiency (low serum ferritin concentrations), the agreement was reasonable for most life stage and gender groups (IOM, 2001). If planners chose to reduce the prevalence of dietary inadequacy (and, by inference, the prevalence of inadequate nutritional status), this could be done using the methods described in Chapter 3 of this report.

In other cases, however, errors in estimating dietary intake make it difficult to use dietary intake data to plan diets with acceptable levels of inadequacy. This is especially true for vitamin E. Food composition data need to be updated for this nutrient, and dietary intakes are frequently underestimated due to underreporting (which may be particularly problematic for fat, a major carrier of vitamin E) (Mertz et al., 1991). Data from NHANES III suggest that the majority of adults aged 31 to 50 had apparently inadequate dietary intakes (IOM, 2000b), leaving the impression that diets must be planned with additional vitamin E to meet the requirements for the population. However, examination of the serum α-tocopherol distributions in NHANES III reveals that fewer than 5 percent had plasma concentrations below the 12 μmol/L (516 μg/dL) used to set the EAR. Thus, for vitamin E, it is clear that the apparent prevalence of dietary inadequacy does not correspond to the prevalence of inadequate nutritional status as assessed biochemically. Thus, when choosing a planning goal, especially when planning for groups, planners need to consider the limitations of the dietary intake data, the consequences of not meeting the criterion used to determine the EAR, the results of available biochemical data, and the goals of dietary planning for specific situations.

As indicated earlier, a nutrient will usually have a Tolerable Upper Intake Level and either an EAR and RDA or an Adequate Intake (AI). However, for energy and the macronutrients, this is not always the case. For example, no DRIs have been set for total fat for individuals over 1 year of age. Instead, an Acceptable Macronutrient Distribution Range of 20 to 35 percent of energy from dietary fat is recommended for adults to minimize risk of adverse health outcomes. For energy, no DRIs have been set—an estimate of the total energy expenditure associated with an individual's gender, age, height, weight, and physical activity level is used.

Uncertainty of Dietary Intake Estimates

Another source of error that has potentially profound implications for dietary assessment and planning is the accuracy of self-reported dietary intakes. A variety of study designs has been employed to examine the accuracy of dietary assessment techniques to measure individuals' true energy intakes over defined time periods. The weight of evidence from this extensive literature indicates that a sizeable proportion of individuals systematically misreport their intakes, with the tendency toward underreporting. In a now classic study by Mertz and colleagues (1991), the usual energy intake of

266 adults (estimated from 7 to 35 days' worth of food records) was determined to be insufficient to maintain body weight in 81 percent of subjects. The average discrepancy between self-reported energy intake and the intake required for weight maintenance was 700 kcal. More recently, self-reports of dietary intake have been compared to energy expenditure measured by doubly labeled water, on the assumption that energy expenditure is equivalent to intake in situations of energy balance. Such comparisons have typically revealed substantial underreporting of intakes, even when changes in body stores during the study period are taken into account (Bandini et al., 1990; Black et al., 1993; Johnson et al., 1998; Kaczkowski et al., 2000; Martin et al., 1996; Prentice et al., 1986; Tomoyasu et al., 1999). Furthermore, although the nature and sources of measurement error are known to vary across dietary assessment methods, the problem of underreporting appears to be pervasive irrespective of whether food records, dietary recalls, diet histories, or food frequency questionnaires are used to assess intake (Black et al., 1991; Sawaya et al., 1996).

Self-reports of dietary intake have also been compared to estimates of energy expenditure based on factorial methods, although at the individual level, this method yields a less precise estimate of energy expenditure than the doubly labeled water technique. Typically, reported energy intake (EI) is expressed as a ratio of estimated basal metabolic rate (BMR_{est}), based on age, sex, self-reported or measured body weight, and possibly height. A variety of approaches to evaluating the adequacy of EI/BMR_{est} can be found in the literature. Goldberg and colleagues (1991) have proposed a method to estimate a minimum plausible EI/BMR_{est} by applying a series of assumptions that take into account within-person variation in energy intake, random error in the estimation of an individual's basal metabolic rate based on the predictive equation used, and variation in an individual's physical activity level. When these methods have been applied to population-based dietary survey data, comparisons indicate that 10 to 50 percent of respondents may be underreporting their food (energy) intakes (Black et al., 1991; Briefel et al., 1997; Johansson et al., 1998; Stallone et al., 1997).

While the underreporting of energy intakes appears well documented, it is unclear how this affects the accuracy of self-reported *nutrient* intakes. Research into this question is limited by the absence of reliable reference biomarkers for intakes of many nutrients. Studies in which the assessment of self-reported energy intake using the doubly labeled water method has been combined with the measurement of urinary nitrogen excretion to assess self-reported protein intake suggest that energy intake may be more prone to under-estimation than protein intake (Larsson et al., 2002). Importantly, these findings imply that all nutrients are not proportionally under-reported; rather, particular foods or classes of foods must be selectively underreported. When the reported intakes by individuals classed as energy underreporters have been compared to those whose energy intakes appear more plausible, underreporters have often been found to report a lower percentage of energy from fat (Becker and Welten, 2001; Becker et al., 1999; Briefel et al., 1997; Goris et al., 2000). Such comparisons have also indicated lower reported consumption of particular classes of foods among under-reporters (Becker and Welten, 2001; Krebs-Smith et al., 2000). How much one can infer about the nature of underreporting from these studies hinges on the validity of the assumption that underreporters' dietary patterns are the same as those not deemed to be under-reporting. Nonetheless, it would appear overly simplistic to assume that the nutrient intakes of individuals who systematically under-report their energy intakes are underreported to the same degree.

The implications of underreporting for dietary assessment and planning are profound given the need to rely on self-reported dietary intakes for information about usual intake patterns. Because individuals' intakes of energy and nutrients are intertwined, the systematic underestimation of true usual energy intakes for some proportion of the population is likely to mean an underestimation of nutrient intakes as well. This is illustrated in a recent analysis of data from a Swedish population survey in which the proportion of individuals with nutrient intakes below the average requirement decreased substantially when individuals reporting "implausibly or dubiously low energy intakes" (defined as $EI/BMR_{est} < 1.10$ and 1.10 to 1.34, respectively, with EI estimated from a 7-day food record) were excluded from the analysis (Becker and Welten, 2001).

Planners are currently limited as to what they can do to correct problems of underreporting. The application of EI/BMR_{est} thresholds to identify underreporters can be problematic, given the need to make assumptions about individuals' usual physical activity levels (often in the absence of good measures of physical activity) and the error inherent in estimates of BMR (an error that is compounded when BMR is calculated using self-reported weight and height). Further, it cannot be assumed that all those with reported energy intakes above the chosen EI/BMR_{est} threshold have accurately reported their intakes. Even if underreporters are somehow identi-fied, the exclusion of their data from population-level assessments of nutrient adequacy clearly threatens the ability to generalize assessment results to the population as a whole. This is because it cannot be assumed that the diets of individuals identified as underreporters are identical to those not so identified.

Well-accepted, validated methods to statistically correct for the effects of underreporting on the estimated distribution of usual intakes are presently lacking. The statistical procedures proposed to adjust intake distributions for within-person variation in intake (e.g., NRC, 1986; Nusser et al., 1996) do not correct for systematic errors in reporting. Application of the residual method of energy adjustment (Willett and Stampfer, 1986) to nutrient distributions has been proposed as one means to reduce the bias associated with energy underreporting without excluding the data of underreporters in some kinds of epidemiological analyses (Stallone et al., 1997). This adjustment method, however, does not provide an appropriate correction of underreporting for dietary intake data to be used in assessment and planning applications of the DRIs. Energy adjustment methods cannot eliminate bias due to selective underreporting of foods; instead these methods effectively "assume" that nutrients have been underreported in direct proportion to energy. Further, energy adjustment does not provide corrected estimates of absolute intake. Thus, energy-adjusted data are not useful in assessments of nutrient adequacy.

In summary, energy underreporting is clearly a serious problem in dietary surveys; it limits the accuracy with which planners can estimate usual energy and nutrient intakes in population groups of interest. Given the current absence of inexpensive, validated methods to readily identify underreporting in dietary intake surveys and statistical methods to correct for underreporting in self-reported energy and nutrient intakes, planners are severely limited in their ability to address this problem.

This problem not only highlights the importance of employing thorough, standardized procedures to collect dietary data, but it also flags the urgent need for more research into statistical methods to analyze and adjust for underreporting in self-reported intake data. In interpreting the results of dietary assessments prior to determining planning goals, planners should look to other sources of data on nutritional status (e.g., anthropometric, clinical, or biochemical assessments) for corroborating evidence. In interpreting dietary assessment results, planners may also find it useful to estimate the extent of energy underreporting in their data by applying factorial methods to compare reported energy intakes with estimates of energy expenditure. However, the crudeness of these estimates should be recognized. Until better methods of identification and adjustment are developed, it is not recommended that data adjustments be undertaken.

Planners can use dietary intake data from national surveys, but should remain aware of the inaccuracies of the data when setting intake goals based on the DRIs and assessing achievement of those goals.

2

Using Dietary Reference Intakes in Planning Diets for Individuals

SUMMARY

The goal of planning a diet for an individual is to achieve a low probability of inadequacy while not exceeding the Tolerable Upper Intake Level (UL) for each nutrient. The Recommended Dietary Allowance (RDA) or Adequate Intake (AI) is used as the target nutrient intake for individuals, and planners should realize that there is no recognized benefit of usual intakes in excess of these levels. Food-based nutrition education tools are regularly used to help an individual plan a healthy diet. However, as a result of the evaluation of new data regarding nutrient requirements presented in the Dietary Reference Intake reports, some nutrition education tools (e.g., the U.S. Food Guide Pyramid and Canada's Food Guide to Healthy Eating) may require revision to remain current. The DRIs are one of several criteria that should be considered when updating such tools.

Assuming that current nutrition education tools have been evaluated to determine if they are consistent with the new reference intakes for nutrients, individuals who wish to plan nutritionally adequate diets for themselves can review their usual intakes with one of the food guides. Food labels can be used to help choose foods that will make up a healthful diet. Individuals can further plan their intakes to be consistent with dietary guidelines (e.g., *Dietary Guidelines for Americans* [USDA/HHS, 2000], *Canada's Guidelines for Healthy Eating* [Health Canada, 1990a]). Gaps or excesses identified can then be remedied by planning to alter the type or amount of foods selected from the various food groups, by using fortified foods, or if necessary, by using nutrient supplements.

INTRODUCTION

The Dietary Reference Intakes (DRIs) are used to establish goals in planning diets for individuals. This may include: (1) providing guidance to healthy individuals who are concerned about meeting their nutrient needs, (2) counseling those with special lifestyle considerations (e.g., athletes and vegetarians) or those requiring therapeutic diets, (3) formulating diets for research purposes, and (4) developing food-based dietary guidance for individuals. This chapter focuses on planning diets for normal healthy individuals. Other situations, including planning therapeutic diets, are addressed in Chapter 6.

Planning diets for individuals involves two steps. First, nutrient goals must be set that are appropriate, taking into account various factors that may have an impact upon nutrient needs. Figure 2-1 provides an algorithm for this process. In this chapter the goal for individual planning is to ensure that the diet *as eaten* has an acceptably low probability of nutrient inadequacy while simultaneously minimizing the risk of nutrient excess. This goal is achieved with

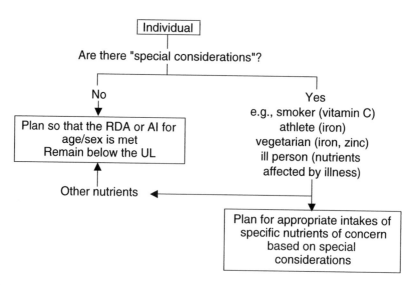

FIGURE 2-1 Schematic decision tree for planning diets for individuals.

diets that meet the recommended intakes (Recommended Dietary Allowance or Adequate Intake) without exceeding the Tolerable Upper Intake Level. Observed intakes may have a high probability of being inadequate or excessive on any given day, but a low probability over time.

When comparing observed intakes to nutrient goals, planners need to be conscious of the errors associated with brief assessments of dietary intake. It is very difficult to obtain accurate estimates of individuals' usual nutrient intakes because intakes typically vary so much from one day to the next. Dietary intakes assessed by multiple 24-hour recalls, dietary records, or quantitative diet histories provide the strongest bases for quantitative assessments of nutrient adequacy, but no method is without error. A full discussion of the uncertainty associated with estimates of an individual's usual intake derived from these methods can be found in the DRI report on dietary assessment (IOM, 2000a). Food frequency questionnaires are not recommended for use in assessments of nutrient adequacy because they have not been found to yield sufficiently accurate estimates of individuals' usual intakes of specific nutrients.

The second step in planning a diet for an individual is to develop a dietary plan that the individual will consume. While the art of crafting appropriate dietary patterns and counseling individuals to achieve them is beyond the scope of this report, information is provided on how to use the DRIs to accomplish these tasks.

SETTING APPROPRIATE NUTRIENT GOALS

As explained in Chapter 1, Dietary Reference Intakes (DRIs) consist of four types of reference intakes that are used to assess and plan diets of individuals and groups: the Estimated Average Requirement (EAR), the Recommended Dietary Allowance (RDA), the Adequate Intake (AI), and the Tolerable Upper Intake Level (UL). The EAR is *not* used as a goal in planning individual diets. By definition, a diet planned to provide the EAR of a nutrient would have a 50 percent likelihood of not meeting an individual's requirement, and this is an unacceptable degree of risk for the individual. What follows is an examination of the RDA, AI, and UL as the three reference intakes related to planning diets for individuals.

Recommended Dietary Allowance

A major goal of dietary planning for individuals is to achieve an acceptably low probability of nutrient inadequacy for a given individual. At the same time, the planner must consider whether increasing an individual's intake beyond its customary level will result in any recognizable benefit. At low levels of intake, the probability of benefit associated with an increase in intake levels is high, but as intake levels rise above the EAR, the probability of benefit of an increased intake diminishes. Planning a diet for an individual that is likely to meet his or her requirement for a nutrient is complicated by the fact that the individual's requirement is almost never known. Most individuals have requirements close to the average requirement for individuals of their sex and age, and the best estimate of an individual's requirement is thus the EAR. However, again by definition, half the individuals in a group have requirements that exceed the EAR. Accordingly, an intake at the level of the EAR would be associated with an unacceptably high risk (50 percent) of not meeting an individual's requirement and would not be suitable as a goal for planning. As intake increases above the EAR, the risk of inadequacy decreases from 50 percent and reaches 2 to 3 percent at the RDA. Thus, the probability of inadequacy is very low for individuals with intakes at the RDA. However, the probability that a given individual will benefit from an increase in intake also decreases to the same extent, and is near zero (less than 2 to 3 percent) when intake increases above the RDA.

The new RDAs may be used as the targets for planning nutrient intakes that result in acceptably low probability of inadequacy for the individual. The RDA is intended to encompass the normal biological variation in the nutrient requirements of individuals. It is set at a level that meets or exceeds the actual nutrient requirements of 97 to 98 percent of individuals in a given life stage and gender group. This level of intake, at which there is a 2 to 3 percent probability of the individual not meeting his or her requirement, has traditionally been adopted as the appropriate reference when planning for individuals. It should be noted that selecting this intake level was, and continues to be, judgmental.

When counseling an individual, it is important to consider whether any recognizable benefit will be achieved if the individual's current intake level is increased. The likelihood of recognizable benefit must be weighed against the costs (monetary and otherwise) likely to be incurred in increasing this intake. An intake level could be chosen at which the risk to the individual is either higher or lower than the 2 to 3 percent level of risk that is inherent in the definition of the RDA.

When other levels are chosen they should be explicitly justified. For example, for a woman between the ages of 19 and 30 years, the

RDA for iron is 18 mg, and is set to cover the needs of women with the highest menstrual blood losses. A particular woman might feel that her menstrual losses were light. Accordingly, she may be willing to accept a 10 percent risk of not meeting her requirements, and thus would have as her goal consumption of only 13 mg of iron/day (see Appendix I in the DRI micronutrient report [IOM, 2001]).

Adequate Intake

An AI is set when scientific evidence is not sufficient to establish an EAR and RDA. Under these circumstances the AI is the target that is used for planning individual diets. Although greater uncertainty exists in determining the probability of inadequacy for a nutrient with an AI than for a nutrient with an RDA, the AI provides a useful basis for planning. However, the probability of inadequacy associated with a failure to achieve the AI is unknown. Unlike a nutrient with an EAR and an RDA, it is not possible to select a level of intake relative to the AI with a known probability of inadequacy.

AIs are set in a variety of ways, as described elsewhere (i.e., IOM, 1997, 1998a, 2000b, 2001, 2002a). But in general they are the observed mean or median nutrient intakes by groups of presumably healthy individuals, or they are based on a review of data derived from both dietary and experimental approaches (e.g., the AIs for calcium and vitamin D [IOM, 1997]). Regardless of how an AI was established, intake at the level of the AI is likely to meet or exceed an individual's requirement, although the possibility that it could fail to meet the requirements of some individuals cannot be discounted.

Tolerable Upper Intake Level

A UL also is provided for many nutrients. The UL is the highest level of chronic daily nutrient intake that is likely to pose no risk of adverse health effects to almost all individuals in the specified life stage and gender group. In general, intakes from food, supplements, and other sources (such as water) should be planned so that the UL is not exceeded. The UL is not a recommended level of intake, but an amount that can be tolerated biologically, with no apparent risk of adverse effects, by almost everyone. Risk to the individual is minimized by diets and practices that provide levels of nutrients below the UL, and thus when planning individual diets, the UL should not be exceeded.

For most nutrients, intakes at or above the UL would rarely be attained from unfortified food alone. For example, the intake of a 31-year-old woman who consumed 3.0 mg of vitamin B_6 was at the 99th percentile of the intakes from food sources reported in the 1994–1996 Continuing Survey of Food Intakes by Individuals (CSFII) in the United States (IOM, 1998a). Her RDA is 1.3 mg/day, and the UL is 100 mg/day. If this same woman decreased her intake to 1.43 mg/day, it would be similar to the 50th percentile of intakes in the CSFII. In either case, her intake would be above the RDA and well below the UL. Even if she added a serving of a highly fortified cereal that contained 2.0 mg of vitamin B_6 per serving to her intake each day, her usual intake would still be well below the UL.

As reported in the CSFII, few individuals had intakes from foods that exceeded the UL. However, since these data were collected, fortification of foods in the United States has increased. In addition, these data did not capture supplement usage. Therefore, it is probable that current intake levels of vitamin B_6 and other nutrients from food sources alone might be higher than those reported in the CSFII.

Close attention to intake from highly concentrated sources of nutrients, such as highly fortified foods or supplements (particularly high-dose single nutrient supplements or high-potency multiple-nutrient supplements) may be warranted for some individuals. For some nutrients, total intake may exceed the UL, especially if a person consumes large amounts from supplements and also has a high intake from food sources. For example, if the same 31-year-old woman, in addition to her diet (the 99th percentile of B_6 intake of 3.0 mg/day), consumed a high-potency single supplement capsule of vitamin B_6 that provided 80 mg/day, her total intake would be 83 mg/day. This amount greatly exceeds the RDA of 1.3 mg/day and approaches the UL of 100 mg/day. If she consumed two supplement capsules per day, her intake would exceed the UL and she would be at potential risk of sensory neuropathy, the adverse effect used to set the UL for vitamin B_6.

Suppose that the same woman consumed a high-potency single supplement of zinc that provided 25 mg/day in addition to her daily dietary intake of 10 mg. Her total zinc intake would be 35 mg/day, which exceeds the RDA of 8 mg/day and approaches the UL of 40 mg/day. If she also consumed a fortified cereal with 100 percent of the Daily Value for zinc (15 mg), the UL would be exceeded. Careful attention must be given when planning diets for individuals consuming high-dose supplements or multiple sources of fortified foods so that total intake does not exceed the UL. There is no documented advantage to intakes that exceed the RDA or AI for healthy persons.

PLANNING FOR ENERGY INTAKES OF INDIVIDUALS

The underlying objective of planning for energy is similar to planning for nutrients—to attain an acceptably low risk of inadequacy and of excess. The approach to planning for energy, however, differs substantially from planning for other nutrients. When planning for individuals for nutrients such as vitamins, minerals, and protein, one plans for a low probability of inadequacy by meeting the Recommended Dietary Allowance (RDA) or Adequate Intake (AI), and a low probability of excess by remaining below the Tolerable Upper Intake Level (UL). Even though intakes at or above the RDA or AI are almost certainly above an individual's requirement, and thus would have little or no likelihood of benefit, there are no adverse effects to the individual of consuming an intake above his or her requirement, provided intake remains below the UL.

The situation for energy is quite different. The best way to assess and plan for energy intake of individuals is to consider the healthfulness of their body weights (or body mass index [BMI]) because with energy there is an obvious adverse effect to individuals who consume intakes above their requirements—over time, weight gain occurs. This difference is reflected in the fact that there is no RDA for energy, as it would be inappropriate to recommend an intake that exceeded the requirement (and would lead to weight gain) of 97 to 98 percent of individuals. Instead, equations have been developed that reflect the total energy expenditure (TEE) as estimated from doubly labeled water data and associated with an individual's sex, age, height, weight, and physical activity level. The product of these equations is termed an estimated energy requirement (EER) (IOM, 2002a).

Although different equations were developed for normal-weight and overweight individuals, because they are quite similar, it is recommended that the equations for normal-weight individuals be used for all individuals (IOM, 2002a). All equations predict total energy expenditure and, by definition, the intake required to maintain an individual's current weight and activity level. They were not designed, for example, to lead to weight loss in overweight individuals. However, just as is the case with other nutrients, energy needs vary from one individual to another, even though their characteristics may be similar. This variability is reflected in the standard deviation (SD) of the requirement estimate, which allows for estimating the range within which the individual's requirements could vary. Note that this does not imply that an individual would maintain energy balance at any intake within this range; it simply indicates how variable requirements could be among those with similar characteristics.

For example, the equation for the EER (IOM, 2002a) for normal-weight women 19 to 50 years of age is:

$$\text{EER (kcal)} = 354.1 - (6.91 \times \text{age [y]}) + \text{physical activity coefficient} \times (9.36 \times \text{weight [kg]} + 726 \times \text{height [m]})$$

This equation can be applied to a 33-year-old woman, 1.63 m in height and weighing 55 kg (BMI = 20.8 kg/m²), whose activity is equivalent to walking about 2 mi/day (this level of activity would be categorized as "low active," and the physical activity coefficient for this activity level is 1.12). Her estimated energy requirement would be calculated as:

$$\text{EER (kcal)} = 354.1 - (6.91 \times 33) + 1.12 \times (9.36 \times 55 + 726 \times 1.63) = 2,028$$

This value of 2,028 kcal represents the average energy requirement of women with her specified characteristics (age, height, weight, and activity level). The SD of the EER is estimated as 70 percent of the standard error of the fit of the regression equation (IOM, 2002a). In this example, the SD of the EER would be 160 kcal. The range within which a given woman's energy requirement likely falls (e.g., the 95 percent confidence interval) would be 2,028 ± (2 × 160 kcal), or between 1,708 and 2,348 kcal/day.

It should be emphasized that usual energy intakes are highly correlated with energy expenditure. This means that most people who have access to enough food will consume an amount of energy very close to what they expend, and as a result, maintain their weight within relatively narrow limits over reasonable periods of time. Any changes in weight that do occur usually reflect small imbalances in intake over expenditure accumulated over a long period of time. For normal individuals who are weight-stable, at a healthy weight, and performing at least the minimal recommended amount of total activity, their energy expenditure (and recommended intake) is their usual energy intake. This also applies to maintaining current weight and activity level in overweight individuals. Thus, if one knew an individual's usual energy intake, one would plan to maintain it rather than calculate the EER to obtain an estimate. In most situations, however, the usual energy intakes of individuals are not known, so the equations for TEE are useful planning tools.

Using the Estimated Energy Requirement to Maintain Body Weight in an Individual

When the planning goal is to maintain body weight in an individual with specified characteristics (age, height, weight, and activity level), an initial planning estimate for energy intake is provided by the equation for TEE of an individual with those characteristics. By definition the estimate would be expected to underestimate the true energy expenditure 50 percent of the time, and to overestimate it 50 percent of the time, leading to corresponding changes in body weight. This indicates that monitoring body weight would be required when using the equations to estimate individual energy expenditure. For example, if one was enrolling subjects in a study in which it was important to maintain body weight with a specified activity level, one might begin by feeding each individual the amount of energy estimated using the equation for their EER. Body weight would be closely monitored over time, and the amount of energy provided to each individual would be adjusted up or down from the EER as required to maintain body weight.

Planning for Macronutrient Distribution

In addition to planning a diet that meets an individual's energy requirements and has a low probability of nutrient inadequacy and potential risk of excess, an individual's intake of macronutrients (e.g., carbohydrate, fat, and protein) should be planned so that carbohydrate, total fat, n-6 and n-3 polyunsaturated fatty acids, and protein are within their respective acceptable ranges (IOM, 2002a). For example, consider the 33-year-old, low-active woman discussed previously, who had an EER of approximately 2,000 kcal. The ranges within which her macronutrient intakes should fall are shown in Table 2-1.

DEVELOPING DIETARY PLANS

Once appropriate nutrient intake goals have been identified for the individual, these must be translated into a dietary plan that is acceptable to the individual. This is most frequently accomplished using nutrient-based food guidance systems.

TABLE 2-1 Distribution of Macronutrient Intake Using the Acceptable Macronutrient Distribution Range for a 33-Year-Old, Low-Active Woman

Macronutrient	Acceptable Macronutrient Distribution Range (% of energy)[a]	Range of Macronutrient Intake for Energy Requirement of ~2000 kcal (g)
Carbohydrate	45–65	225–325
Protein	10–35	50–175
Total fat	20–35	44–78
n-6 Polyunsaturated fatty acids	5–10	11–22
n-3 Polyunsaturated fatty acids	0.6–1.2	1.3–2.7
Added sugars	< 25	< 500 kcal

[a] Source: IOM (2002a).

Nutrient-Based Food Guidance Systems in the United States and Canada

Dietary reference standards (e.g., the former Recommended Dietary Allowances [RDAs] in the United States and the Recommended Nutrient Intakes [RNIs] in Canada) have been used to provide food-based dietary guidance in many ways, including through development of national food guides and dietary guidelines for healthy populations and as a basis for information on food and supplement labels. Dietary guidance systems and food composition tables are the most universally accessible sources of nutrition information available to practitioners and laypersons. Practitioners may also use many other sources of nutrition information for individual planning (such as new information in the scientific literature or information on disease prevention from professional associations).

In practice, guidance about food choices, such as the U.S. Food Guide Pyramid or Canada's Food Guide to Healthy Eating, are widely used. These guides recommend that users select the appropriate amount of food for their age, sex, physiological status, body size, and physical activity level from among a range of servings from several different food groups. The intent is that over a period of days to weeks, varied choices within each group allow recommended intakes of nutrients to be attained. The former RDAs and RNIs were two of the major elements from which these food guidance systems were developed; future revisions will undoubtedly consider the new Dietary Reference Intakes (DRIs). Thus, reference standards for nutrients are implicitly used in planning individual diets when food guides are used.

The following sections present a brief summary of the ways that nutrient recommendations have been used in food guides and food labels. Appendix B provides a more detailed description.

Food Guides in the United States and Canada

Both the Food Guide Pyramid (Figure 2-2) and the Food Guide to Healthy Eating (Figure 2-3) are guides for healthy persons to achieve adequate total nutrient intakes from food sources. Adjustments in intakes due to varying requirements (e.g., age, sex, physiological status) are accomplished with these tools by modifying the number of servings consumed. In these systems, foods within a group are assumed to have particular and fairly similar nutrient profiles, and the specified serving sizes are based in part on an amount that would provide comparable levels of key nutrients from

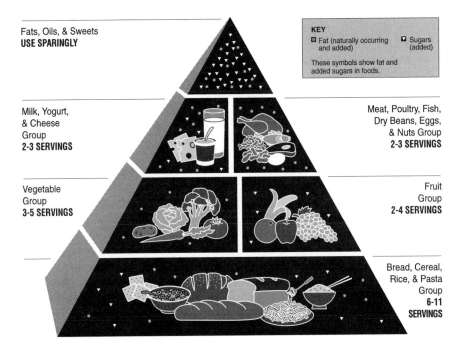

FIGURE 2-2 U.S. Food Guide Pyramid.
SOURCE: USDA (1992).

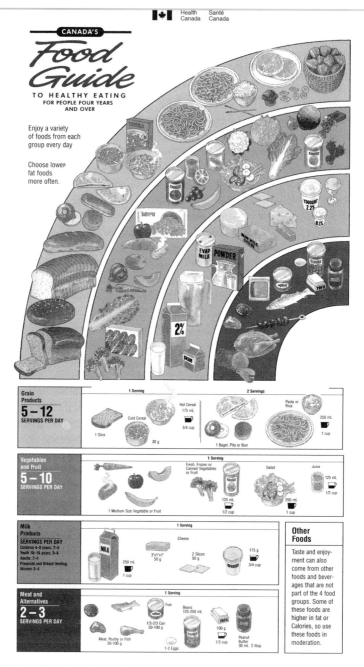

FIGURE 2-3 Canada's Food Guide to Healthy Eating.
SOURCE: Health Canada (1991).

foods within the group. For example, each serving in the "meat and alternatives" group is a good source of protein. One serving of any of the alternatives in this group would have approximately the same amount of protein. As indicated earlier, the design of food guidance systems is that, over a period of time (days or weeks), individuals who consume the recommended number of servings from each food group, and who choose a variety of foods within each group, will obtain the recommended intakes for all nutrients.

As an example, consider an active 22-year-old pregnant woman who receives dietary counseling. Using the Food Guide Pyramid as a guide to achieve the recommended intakes of nutrients, her meal pattern would include a minimum of three servings (7 oz) of protein-rich foods, three servings of dairy products, two servings of fruits, and three servings of vegetables (focusing on foods rich in folate, vitamin C, and β-carotene), and seven servings from the bread, cereal, rice, and pasta group. Additional servings of foods from these groups and from the tip of the pyramid would be added if needed to meet energy requirements. From this the nutritionist would develop a menu plan and an example of food choices based on the above dietary pattern.

Table 2-2 is an example of planning a day's menu using the Food Guide Pyramid. Table 2-3 compares its nutrient content to the current RDAs or Adequate Intakes (AIs) for nutrients. It can be seen that the sample day's menu exceeds intake recommendations for all nutrients, even though it is for only one day. It is important to emphasize that food choices within this menu pattern would vary, and the intake from the one sample day will not accurately reflect the average intake over several days. For example, the average intake of nutrients provided by the sample day's menu in amounts substantially above the RDA could decrease (e.g., the sample menu provides vitamin A in amounts well above the RDA because carrots, a concentrated source of the provitamin A carotenoid, β-carotene, were included). It is expected that varied food choices within the menu pattern would allow average intake to meet recommendations for most nutrients and energy needs.

Those who use food guides to plan menus for individuals must recognize that when new reference intakes for nutrients are developed, there is an unavoidable time lag before the guides can be assessed to determine whether they support the new nutrient reference standards. When new reference intakes have changed considerably from previous standards, a food guide may not be appropriate. For example, the new RDAs for vitamin A (IOM, 2001), while somewhat lower than the previous standards, specify the use of

TABLE 2-2 Sample Planning Menu for a Prenatal Client Aged 22 Years Based on the Food Guide Pyramid

Breakfast	Lunch	Mid-Afternoon Snack	Dinner	Evening Snack
$3/4$ cup orange juice (FG)	2 oz tuna fish (PRG)	5 wheat crackers (BCG)	1 cup skim milk (DG)	1 cup yogurt (nonfat) (DG)
1 cup fortified wheat cereal with raisins (BCG)	1 tsp mayonnaise (FSG)	2 tbsp peanut butter (PRG)	4 oz roasted chicken breast (PRG)	$1/2$ cup fresh blueberries (FG)
1 slice mixed grain toast (BCG)	2 slices whole wheat bread (BCG) (with lettuce and tomato)	1 apple (FG)	1 cup cooked long grain rice (BCG)	$1/4$ cup dry roasted almonds (PRG)
1 tsp margarine (FSG)	$1/2$ cup cooked carrots (VG)	1 cup skim milk (DG)	$1/2$ cup cooked spinach (VG)	
1 tbsp jelly (FSG)	1 glass sweetened iced tea		1 cup tossed salad (VG)	
1 cup skim milk (DG)			2 tbsp low-fat French dressing (FSG)	

NOTE: Nutrient analysis was performed using Nutritionist Five, First DataBank, Inc. 2000. FG = fruit group, BCG = bread and cereal group (bread, cereal, rice, and pasta), FSG = fat and sweet group (fats, oils, and sweets), DG = dairy group (milk, yogurt, and cheese), PRG= protein-rich group (meat, poultry, fish, dry beans, eggs, nuts), VG = vegetable group.

retinol activity equivalents (RAE) rather than retinol equivalents (RE) when calculating or reporting the amount of total vitamin A in mixed or plant foods. An RAE gives the β-carotene:retinol equivalency ratio as 12:1, versus the former equivalency of 6:1 (NRC, 1989). The increased ratio means that a larger amount of β-carotene is needed to meet the vitamin A requirement for individuals who rely on plant sources of this vitamin in their diet. Therefore, newer food guides may need to reflect an increase in the amount of darkly colored, carotene-rich fruits and vegetables needed to provide vitamin A in the diet.

Consideration should be given to the new DRIs when food guides are updated. In the interim, dietetic practitioners who plan diets should familiarize themselves with the nutrient intake recommen-

TABLE 2-3 Comparison of Nutrient Intake with Current Recommended Intake, Based on a Sample Planning Menu (Table 2-2)

Nutrient	Planned Intake	RDA or AI for Pregnancy[a]	Planned Intake as % of RDA or AI
Energy (kcal)	2,363	2,365 EER[b]	
Protein (g)	131	71[c]	185
Carbohydrate (g)	320	175	183
Vitamin A (μg RAE)[d]	2,253	770 μg RAE	293
Vitamin C (mg)	140	85	165
Vitamin E (mg α-tocopherol)[e]	15	15	100
Thiamin (mg)	1.9	1.4	135
Riboflavin (mg)	3.5	1.4	250
Niacin (mg)	44	18	244
Vitamin B$_6$ (mg)	3.0	1.9	158
Folate (μg)	606	600 μg DFE[f]	101
Vitamin B$_{12}$ (μg)	8.2	2.6	315
Calcium (mg)	1,841	1,000	184
Copper (mg)	1.9	1.0	190
Iron (mg)	41	27	152
Magnesium (mg)	649	350	185
Phosphorus (mg)	2,505	700	358
Zinc (mg)	14	11	127

[a] RDA = Recommended Dietary Allowance, AI = Adequate Intake.
[b] Estimated Energy Requirement (EER) = 354.1 − (6.91 × 22) + 1.27 × (9.36 × 54 + 726 × 1.65) + 0 (pregnancy energy deposition for first trimester) = 2,365 kcal.
[c] Protein = 46 g/day + 25 g/day of additional protein during pregnancy.
[d] Database values for vitamin A in retinol equivalents (RE) were converted to retinol activity equivalents (RAE). For retinol, 1 RE = 1 RAE. For carotenoids, 1 RE = 0.5 RAE.
[e] Nineteen α-tocopherol equivalents (α-TE) × 0.8 mg = 15.2 mg α-tocopherol, where 0.8 is the ratio of α-tocopherol to α-TE.
[f] 1 μg dietary folate equivalent (DFE) = 1 μg food folate.

dations that have changed substantially, examine existing tools, and modify methods as necessary to ensure that these targets are met.

Fortified Foods

Fortified and enriched foods have the advantage of providing additional sources of certain nutrients that might otherwise be present only in low amounts in some food sources. Therefore, they are helpful in planning diets to reduce the probability of inadequacy of specific nutrients. In addition, they may afford the opportunity to add nutrients in highly bioavailable forms, as is the case with folate- and vitamin B_{12}-fortified foods.

The fortification of foods is undertaken for public health reasons. For example, in the United States and Canada, iodized salt; cereal grains fortified with thiamin, riboflavin, niacin, iron, and folate; and vitamin D-fortified milk were intended to reduce the risk of inadequate intakes of those nutrients. Fortification provides a food-based means for increasing intakes of particular nutrients and in some cases can be especially targeted to specific groups at risk of shortfalls in specific nutrients (e.g., infant formulas and infant cereals fortified with iron are useful to meet the high iron needs of older infants and young children).

In addition to fortification initiated by government authorities for public health reasons, independent voluntary fortification undertaken by private industry is also allowed in the United States. Often the amount of a nutrient added during such voluntary fortification may be based on commercial appeal, rather than public health analysis of desirable dietary additions. It is necessary to use highly fortified foods selectively when planning diets so that they contribute to nutrient adequacy without causing excess intakes. Canadian regulations are different and do not permit independent voluntary fortification. (For additional information, see Appendix D.)

Nutrient Supplements

Nutrient supplements provide an additional means of consuming specific nutrients that otherwise might be in short supply. Depending on their formulation, they may consist of single nutrients or a combination of many different vitamins, elements, or other nutrient and nonnutrient ingredients. Doses vary from levels close to the RDA or AI to several times these levels. Supplements are useful when they fill a specific identified nutrient gap that cannot or is not otherwise being met by the individual's food-based dietary intake. For example, it is recommended that women who might become pregnant obtain 400 µg of folic acid from the use of fortified foods or supplements, in addition to obtaining folate from a varied diet. For pregnant women, iron supplements may be suggested to meet needs for this nutrient that are unlikely to be achieved from food sources alone (IOM, 1992). However, there can be disadvantages associated with supplement use. For example, individuals at risk may not adhere to the supplement regimen. In other cases, those who are already consuming the RDA or AI for most nutrients from food sources may use supplements, but they will not achieve any recognized health benefit from consuming more of these nutrients as supplements and may be at risk of excessive intake.

Food and Supplement Labels in the United States and Canada

In the United States, the percent of Daily Values stated on food and supplement labels for vitamins and elements is based on the Reference Daily Intakes (RDI) established by the Food and Drug Administration. In the early 1990s, the term RDI replaced the term "US RDA" for vitamins and elements on food labeling. The current RDI values are the same as the US RDAs that were provided on food labels in the past, which are based on the highest RDA across the various age and gender categories (with the exception of pregnancy and lactation) from the 1968 RDAs (NRC, 1968). Additional RDI values have been added for nutrients for which there were no RDAs in 1968 (e.g., folate). Table 2-4 compares the current RDA or AI to the US RDI. An example of a U.S. food label is shown in Figure 2-4.

In Canada the food and supplement labels are based on the highest RNI for any age and gender group over age 2 from the 1983 Canadian RNIs (Consumer and Corporate Affairs Canada, 1988). Table 2-4 also compares the values used for the food label in Canada with the current RDAs or AIs. Canadian nutrition labeling has recently been revised, and the new label closely resembles the U.S nutrition label. An example of the new Canadian label format is shown in Figure 2-5.

Similar to the previously discussed situation with food guides, food labels also may not reflect the most current nutrient reference standards. Consumers need to be aware of the discrepancies that exist when using the food label information to plan their diets.

Dietary Guidelines in the United States and Canada

The U.S. Dietary Guidelines and Canada's Guidelines for Healthy Eating are designed to provide advice about dietary patterns that promote health and prevent chronic disease in a healthy population (see Appendix B). The dietary guidelines describe food choices that will help individuals meet their recommended intake of nutrients. Like the DRIs, the guidelines apply to diets consumed over several days—not a single day or single meal. Nutrient reference standards are not the primary focus of dietary guidelines, but when selecting healthy food choices based on the guidelines, individuals are more likely to meet recommended intakes of nutrients and to have macronutrient intakes that fall within the acceptable macro-

TABLE 2-4 Comparison of the Recommended Dietary Allowances (RDA) and Adequate Intakes (AI) with Daily Values (DV) for Vitamins and Minerals Used on Food Labels in the United States and Canada

Nutrient	RDA or AI[a]	U.S. Reference Daily Intake (DV)[b]	Canadian DV[c]
Vitamin A (µg)	900 RAE	5,000 IU	1,000 RE
Vitamin C (mg)	90	60	60
Vitamin D (µg)	15	10	5
Vitamin E (mg α-tocopherol)	15	30 IU	10
Thiamin (mg)	1.2	1.5	1.3
Riboflavin (mg)	1.3	1.7	1.6
Niacin (mg)	16	20	23 NE
Vitamin B$_6$ (mg)	1.7	2.0	1.8
Folate (µg)	400	400	220
Vitamin B$_{12}$ (µg)	2.4	6	2
Pantothenic acid (mg)	5	10	7
Biotin (µg)	30	300	—
Choline (mg)	550	—	—
Calcium (mg)	1,300	1,000	1,100
Chromium (µg)	35	120	—
Copper (mg)	0.9	2	—
Fluoride (mg)	4	—	—
Iodine (µg)	150	150	160
Iron (mg)	18	18	14
Magnesium (mg)	420	400	250
Phosphorus (mg)	1,250	1,000	1,100
Selenium (µg)	55	—	—
Zinc (mg)	11	15	9

[a] Highest values for any age/sex category except pregnant/lactating. RAE = retinol activity equivalents.

[b] The U.S. DVs are higher than the recently recommended intakes (RDAs or AIs) for thiamin, riboflavin, niacin, vitamin B$_6$, vitamin B$_{12}$, pantothenic acid, biotin, chromium, copper, and zinc. The DVs are lower for vitamin C, vitamin D, calcium, magnesium, and phosphorus. It is not possible to directly compare vitamin A, vitamin E, and folate because the DV is in International Units (IU) while the RDA is in mg or µg and different bioavailability factors are incorporated into the values. There are three nutrients with an RDA or AI but no DV (choline, fluoride, and selenium).

[c] The Canadian DVs are higher than the RDAs or AIs for thiamin, riboflavin, niacin, vitamin B$_6$, pantothenic acid, and iodine. The DVs are lower for vitamin C, vitamin D, vitamin E, folate, vitamin B$_{12}$, calcium, iron, magnesium, and phosphorus. There are six nutrients with an RDA or AI but no RDI (biotin, choline, chromium, copper, fluoride, and selenium). RE = retinol equivalents, NE = niacin equivalents.

Nutrition Facts

Serving Size 1 cup (228g)
Serving Per Container 2

Amount Per Serving

Calories 250   Calories from Fat 110

	% Daily Value*
Total Fat 12g	**18%**
Saturated Fat 3g	**15%**
Cholesterol 30mg	**10%**
Sodium 470mg	**20%**
Total Carbohydrate 31g	**10%**
Dietary Fiber 0g	**0%**
Sugars 5g	
Protein 5g	

Vitamin A	4%
Vitamin C	2%
Calcium	20%
Iron	4%

* Percent Daily Values are based on a 2,000 calorie diet.
Your Daily Values may be higher or lower depending on
your calorie needs:

	Calories:	2,000	2,500
Total Fat	Less than	65g	80g
Sat Fat	Less than	20g	25g
Cholesterol	Less than	300mg	300mg
Sodium	Less than	2,400mg	2,400mg
Total Carbohydrate		300g	375g
Dietary Fiber		25g	30g

FIGURE 2-4 U.S. food label.
SOURCE: FDA (2000).

nutrient distribution ranges. For example, the U.S. guideline "Let the Pyramid Guide Your Food Choices" promotes dietary nutrient adequacy. The Canadian guideline "Enjoy a Variety of Foods" is based on the principle that foods contain combinations of nutrients and other substances that are needed for good health. Thus, an individual is more likely to meet nutrient needs by eating a variety of foods. The U.S. guidelines also emphasize choosing a variety of grains, especially whole grains, and consuming adequate servings of fruits and vegetables, which provide important nutrients that may be low among some population subgroups (e.g., pregnant women

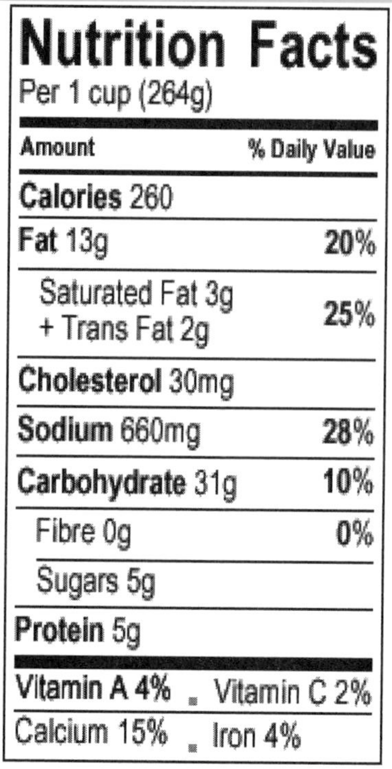

Nutrition Facts
Per 1 cup (264g)

Amount	% Daily Value
Calories 260	
Fat 13g	20%
Saturated Fat 3g + Trans Fat 2g	25%
Cholesterol 30mg	
Sodium 660mg	28%
Carbohydrate 31g	10%
Fibre 0g	0%
Sugars 5g	
Protein 5g	
Vitamin A 4% ▪ Vitamin C 2%	
Calcium 15% ▪ Iron 4%	

FIGURE 2-5 Canadian food label.
SOURCE: Health Canada (2002).

and the elderly). The guidelines state that fruits and vegetables are excellent sources of folate and antioxidant nutrients such as vitamin C, vitamin E, and carotenoids, and thus help to prevent nutrient inadequacy. In addition, high intakes of fruits and vegetables are associated with reduced disease risk and are good sources of phytochemicals. The guidelines also serve to promote the importance of moderation and avoiding excess salt, fat, sugar, and alcoholic beverages. The guidelines, if followed, also ensure moderation in intakes of foods that provide energy but few nutrients.

3

Using Dietary Reference Intakes in Planning Diets for Groups

SUMMARY

The framework for group planning presented in this chapter focuses on the distribution of usual nutrient intakes as the basis for planning. This chapter describes the framework as it applies to planning for groups that are homogeneous in regard to life stage and gender, while Chapter 4 presents an approach to planning for heterogeneous groups.

The overall goal of planning for groups is to achieve usual intakes in the group that meet the requirements of most individuals, but are not excessive. This is accomplished by combining information on the group's nutrient requirements with information on its usual nutrient intakes. This information is used to plan for a usual nutrient intake distribution in which intakes will meet the requirement of all but a specified proportion of the group. This framework importantly shifts the focus of planning away from past practices of using dietary recommendations or Recommended Dietary Allowances to decide what to serve, toward what is ultimately desired in terms of the distribution of usual intakes as measured by actual consumption. To apply the framework presented here, an acceptable prevalence of inadequacy must be defined and the distribution of usual intakes in the group must be estimated. The target usual intake distribution can then be determined by positioning the distribution of usual intakes relative to the Estimated Average Requirement or nutrient requirement distribution so as to achieve the desired prevalence of inadequacy. When positioning the distribution, the prevalence of intakes above the Tolerable Upper Intake Level (UL) also must be considered. Because the goal of planning is to achieve a desired distribution of usual intake, it is clear that to judge the success of the planning activity, assessment must occur. In most situations, planning group diets is an iterative, ongoing effort in which planners set planning goals for usual intake, assess whether the goals are achieved, and then modify their planning procedures accordingly.

GENERAL CONSIDERATIONS

Planning diets for groups is a multistep process. It involves identifying the specific nutritional goals, determining how best to achieve these goals, and, ultimately, assessing if these goals are achieved. Planning the diets of groups also involves multiple components. Planners must decide what foods to purchase, what foods and combinations of foods to offer, how the foods should be prepared, and the quantities to serve. Planners must also recognize that individuals within a group look at what foods are offered and then decide what foods to select and, finally, what foods to eat.

To address all these planning components would be an ambitious effort; many of these issues are not specifically related to using and interpreting the Dietary Reference Intakes (DRIs). This report focuses primarily on the ultimate goal of group planning as achieving a usual intake distribution with a low prevalence of inadequate or excessive intakes. In this chapter, the focus is on planning for groups that are homogeneous in terms of life stage and gender, while Chapter 4 presents an approach to planning for groups that vary in life stage and gender.

In planning diets for groups, planners often adopt broad nutritional goals and then design their programs to offer meals and diets that meet recognized nutritional standards. For example, when deciding how to plan meals for an institution like a boarding school or an assisted living facility, the objective is often to provide food with a given level of nutrients. However, it would be more appropriate to know how much of the offered food is actually consumed and what the resulting distribution of nutrient intakes is likely to be. Unless the distribution of intakes is considered, the amount being offered may not be sufficient for a substantial proportion of the residents to obtain enough of a nutrient to meet their requirements. This approach is also illustrated by some of the national food assistance programs. The objective of the Food Stamp Program, for example, is to provide low-income households with benefits so they can purchase a low-cost, nutritionally adequate diet. However, the current goal is to offer (i.e., make available) an adequate diet, which does not necessarily translate into a low prevalence of inadequate intakes among the eligible households.

The group-feeding framework proposed in this report differs from how many planning applications are currently designed. Because this framework considers the distribution of usual nutrient intakes of the group as the basis for planning, it shifts the focus of planning away from using dietary recommendations in deciding what to offer, to what is ultimately desired in terms of the distribution of usual nutrient intake.

By focusing explicitly on the distribution of nutrient intakes of a group as the goal of group planning, the framework presented below is, in many respects, a new paradigm, and it should be tested before being implemented in large-scale group-feeding situations.

It is important to remember, however, that while planners may have desired nutrient intakes of the group as their ultimate objective, they typically can control only what is offered to individuals in the group. In this proposed framework, therefore, the link between planning and assessment is crucial. That is, since the goal of planning is to achieve a usual intake distribution with a high group prevalence of nutrient adequacy (i.e., an acceptably low group prevalence of inadequacy), then it is clear that to judge the success of the planning activity, assessment must occur.

When planning the diets of population groups, it is important to consider how usual intakes will be *distributed*, not just the mean or median intake. For some planning applications, the goal is to correctly position an intake distribution, but not to intentionally change its shape (see Figure 3-1 as an example of repositioning a distribution). In other situations it may be desirable to change the shape of the intake distribution for one or more nutrients, perhaps by targeting individuals in the tails of the distribution. This chapter first addresses group feeding where changing the shape of the distribution is not an explicit goal, and then discusses the additional challenges of planning intakes for interventions when the goal is to alter some part of the distribution. However, it is very important to keep in mind that any intervention that is designed to affect intakes of all or just some individuals in a group will more than likely result in an intake distribution that differs from the baseline distribution not only in location, but also in shape.

The framework presented in this chapter assumes that the group is large enough so that planning and assessing do not occur at the individual level. That is, one can neither plan for specific individuals within a group nor assess the results of group planning for specific individuals in the group. In some situations, however, it may not be clear whether planners should follow procedures to plan diets for individuals or for groups. Usually the decision is driven by the information available for individuals within the group, as well as by the availability of resources to tailor diets to individual needs.

In group-feeding situations such as the National School Lunch Program, information about individuals is generally not available, and it is clear that group-planning procedures should be used. However, when the characteristics of individuals are well known to planners (e.g., a small group home for children with a variety of physical and developmental disabilities), planning may occur primarily at the individual level. Or, among groups of hospitalized patients, information about individual characteristics is potentially available, but is used only in certain cases. Planners will know whether a given individual is following a therapeutic diet (e.g., cholesterol lowering, diabetic, renal) and will also have access to additional personal information (e.g., age, sex, body size). However, for most patients on nontherapeutic diets, individual information is usually not used in planning—thus, a "hybrid" approach to planning may be adopted in which a group planning approach is used for most patients, while those on therapeutic diets may be planned for as individuals.

It is clear from the above discussion that group-feeding situations can vary considerably, and in some situations, planners may combine elements of group and individual planning. The following discussion, however, focuses only on group planning.

OVERVIEW OF PLANNING FOR NUTRIENT INTAKES OF GROUPS

Planning nutrient intakes for a group is difficult because individuals in a group, even if offered the same meal, vary in the amount and selection of foods that they eat. Planning for group feeding typically focuses on planning for institutional feeding, which includes such settings as residential schools, prisons, military garrisons, hospitals, and nursing homes. By a slight extension, this category of planning also includes many food and nutrition assistance programs such as the Food Stamp Program, child nutrition programs, and emergency food assistance programs.

The underlying principle for group planning is that the resulting distri-

bution of usual nutrient intakes will have a low prevalence of inadequate or excessive intake, as defined by the proportion of individuals in the group with usual intakes less than the Estimated Average Requirement (EAR) or greater than the Tolerable Upper Intake Level (UL).

To explain this framework it is important to review briefly the methods available for assessing the prevalence of inadequate intakes of groups. As discussed in detail in the DRI assessment report (IOM, 2000a), two related methods can be used to estimate the prevalence of inadequate intakes in a group:

1. *Probability approach.* The probability approach involves determining the probability of inadequacy for each usual intake level in the population and then averaging the individual probabilities of inadequacy across the group to obtain an estimate of the group prevalence of inadequacy. This method of dietary assessment depends on two key assumptions: intakes and requirements are independent, and the distribution of requirements is known.

2. *EAR cut-point method.* Under certain conditions, the prevalence of inadequate intakes for a group can be estimated as the proportion of the group with usual intakes less than the EAR. The EAR cut-point method is an approximation of the probability approach and can be used in most situations provided the following assumptions are met: (1) intakes and requirements are independent, (2) the requirement distribution is symmetrical around the EAR, and (3) the variance in intakes is larger than the variance in requirements.

Concept of a Target Usual Nutrient Intake Distribution

Suppose a planner is interested in planning a group diet with a high probability of nutrient adequacy (e.g., such that the prevalence of inadequacy in the group is no more than 2 to 3 percent). Given this targeted prevalence, and assuming that the EAR cut-point method can be used in assessment, the usual intake distribution of the group should be positioned such that only 2 to 3 percent of individuals in the group have usual intakes less than the EAR (see Figure 3-1, Panel B, as an example). To achieve this goal of a low prevalence of nutrient inadequacy, it may be necessary to modify the baseline usual nutrient intake distribution. The change may be as simple as a shift (up or down) of the entire baseline distribution or it may include changes in both the location and the shape of the distribution. In either case, the appropriate changes to the baseline usual nutrient intake distribution are intended to result in the desired distribution of usual intakes. This desired distribution is referred to as the target usual nutrient intake distribution.

The simplest approach to determining the target usual nutrient intake distribution is to shift the baseline distribution, with the assumption that there will be no change in its shape. This is illustrated in Figure 3-1 for a hypothetical nutrient. Panel A shows the baseline usual intake distribution in which the prevalence of inadequate intakes (percentage of the group below the EAR) is about 30 percent. If the planning goal was to attain a prevalence of inadequacy of no more than 2 to 3 percent, the target usual nutrient intake distribution could be achieved by simply shifting the baseline usual intake distribution up, as shown in Panel B.

The appropriate shift (up or down) can be calculated as the additional (or decreased) amount of the nutrient that must be consumed to attain the prevalence of usual intakes below the EAR that is the planning goal. For example, the EAR for zinc for girls 9 to 13 years old is 7 mg/day. Current data from the Third National Health and Nutrition Examination Survey (NHANES III, as reported in IOM, 2001) show that about 10 percent of the girls have usual intakes below the EAR. If the goal were to plan intakes so that only 2 to 3 percent are below the EAR, intakes would have to be increased. When the intervention is designed to increase everyone's usual zinc intake, then the amount of the increase can be calculated as the difference between the current intake at the 2nd to 3rd percentile (which is 6.2 mg/day) and the desired intake at the 2nd to 3rd percentile (the EAR of 7 mg/day); the difference is thus 0.8 mg/day. That means that the distribution of usual intakes needs to shift up by 0.8 mg/day in order to have only 2 to 3 percent of the girls with intakes below the EAR.

The same goal of 97 to 98 percent adequate intakes could, in theory, be achieved by planning an intervention that is designed to increase the usual zinc intake of only those individuals who have low baseline zinc intake levels. However, in most group-planning situations it is not possible to identify who these individuals are, making this type of planning procedure difficult to implement.

The target usual nutrient intake distribution should also be examined to determine if it meets the goal of a low prevalence of potentially excessive intakes. For zinc, the UL for girls 9 to 13 years old is 23 mg/day. The 99th percentile of their current intake distribution is 15.5 mg/day, so even if the distribution is shifted up by 0.8 mg/day, the 99th percentile (16.3 mg/day) is well below the UL.

The Median of the Target Usual Nutrient Intake Distribution

The median of the target usual nutrient intake distribution is a useful summary measure. As will be discussed later in this chapter (see "Planning Menus to Achieve Target Usual Nutrient Intake Distributions"), it may be used as a tool in the menu planning process.

Assuming that the shape of the intake distribution does not change as a result of planning, the median of the target usual nutrient intake distribution is calculated as the median of the current usual intake distribution, plus (or minus) the amount that the distribution needs to shift to make it the target usual nutrient intake distribution.

Figure 3-1 illustrates this concept. In this example, the planning goal is to achieve a distribution of usual intake such that only 2 to 3

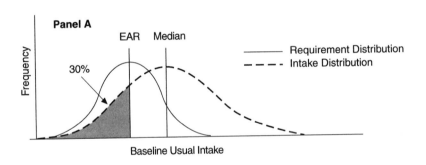

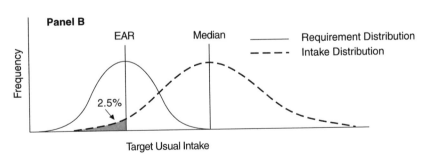

FIGURE 3-1 Concept of a target usual intake distribution. Panel A shows the baseline usual nutrient intake distribution, in which the prevalence of inadequate intake (percentage below Estimated Average Requirement) is about 30 percent. Shifting the baseline distribution up so that the prevalence of inadequate intakes reflects the planning goal (in this example, 2 to 3 percent) attains the target usual nutrient intake distribution (Panel B).

percent of the group has usual intakes below the EAR. The amount that the baseline usual nutrient intake distribution (Panel A) needs to shift so that it becomes the target usual nutrient intake distribution (Panel B) can be determined as the difference between intake at the 2nd to 3rd percentile of the baseline distribution and the EAR. This amount, added to the median of the baseline distribution, defines the median of the target intake distribution. (Under the assumption of normality of the usual intake distribution, the median of the target usual nutrient intake distribution can be calculated directly as the EAR + 2 standard deviations [SD] of intake.) Assuming that the shape of the intake distribution does not change when it is shifted, only 2 to 3 percent of the individuals in the group will have usual intakes less than the EAR when the target distribution is positioned in this manner.

How does the median of the target usual nutrient intake distribution compare with the Recommended Dietary Allowance (RDA)?

The relationship between the median of the target usual nutrient intake distribution and the RDA depends on the selected prevalence of inadequacy. With a prevalence of inadequacy of 2 to 3 percent, the target median intake usually exceeds the RDA.

In the zinc example used above for girls 9 to 13 years of age, the distribution needs to be shifted by an additional 0.8 mg/day. The median of the current zinc distribution for these girls is 9.4 mg/day, so the median of the target usual nutrient intake distribution would be 9.4 + 0.8 = 10.2 mg/day.

The median of a target usual nutrient intake distribution exceeds the RDA because the variance in usual intakes typically exceeds the variance of the requirement. Recall that in the case of a normal distribution of requirements, the RDA equals the EAR + 2 SDs of the *requirement*. However, the target usual nutrient intake distribution (and therefore, its median) is determined based on the variability of *intakes*. In the zinc example, the RDA for girls is 8 mg/day, but the target median intake is 10.2 mg/day. Thus, selection of the RDA levels as the median of the target usual intake distribution is not recommended as it results in a percentage of inadequacy greater than would likely be selected with more careful consideration.

In positioning the distribution of usual intakes relative to the EAR, the same three assumptions delineated earlier as being required to use the EAR cut-point method in the dietary assessment of groups must be satisfied (IOM, 2000a). Later in this chapter, methods are described for estimating the target usual nutrient intake distribution when these assumptions are not valid.

CONSIDERATIONS IN PLANNING FOR A TARGET USUAL NUTRIENT INTAKE DISTRIBUTION

Planning for a target usual nutrient intake distribution involves several considerations, which form the basis of the following discussion. These include:

- estimating the existing or baseline distribution of usual nutrient intake;
- selecting the target prevalence of inadequacy;
- estimating the target usual nutrient intake distribution;
- assessing the feasibility of obtaining the target usual nutrient intake distribution; and
- planning for groups when assumptions of the Estimated Average Requirement cut-point method are violated.

Estimating the Existing or Baseline Distribution of Usual Nutrient Intake

Estimating the target usual nutrient intake distribution requires information about the shape of the existing distribution of usual nutrient intakes. Specifically, the distribution of usual intakes is needed, with the effect of day-to-day variation removed. The between-person variance in usual intakes is typically less than the variance of the observed distribution of intakes in a group, because the latter includes both within-person (day-to-day) variation and between-person (individual-to-individual) variation. Thus, the observed intake distribution must be adjusted to approximate the distribution of true usual intakes in the group.

To estimate the distribution of usual intakes directly for the group of interest, the actual intakes of a representative sample of the group must be assessed over at least two nonconsecutive days or three consecutive days and an adjustment procedure applied (IOM, 2000a). Food frequency questionnaires are not recommended for use in assessments of usual nutrient intakes because of concerns about the accuracy of nutrient intake estimates derived from this approach (see the Dietary Reference Intakes assessment report [IOM, 2000a] for a full discussion of this issue). Rather, intakes should be assessed through the use of 24-hour dietary intake recalls or diet records.

Procedures to adjust observed intake distributions to remove the effect of within-person variation have been developed (IOM, 2000a; NRC, 1986; Nusser et al., 1996). It should be noted, however, that the most appropriate adjustment method depends in part on the size of the group, with the Iowa State University method (Nusser et al., 1996) recommended for large groups, but the National Research Council (NRC, 1986) method perhaps offering advantages in the adjustment of intake distributions for small samples (defined here as groups smaller than 40 to 50 people). A discussion of these methods is presented in Appendix E. Using the adjusted distribution, planners can identify the percentiles of intake that describe the distribution of usual intakes.

In many group-planning activities, a baseline or current usual nutrient intake for the group being planned for may not be available. In these situations it may be possible to approximate the percentiles of usual intake for the target group from existing data on usual intakes for a group with similar characteristics. Distributions of usual nutrient intake derived from general population surveys are presented in appendixes to the DRI reports (IOM, 1997, 1998a, 2000b, 2001, 2002a), and these percentiles of intake may be appropriate for use in some planning activities. Where such secondary sources are used, however, planners must be careful to consider factors in the target group that contribute to between-person variation in usual intakes and verify that the same types of factors are present in the group from which the distribution of usual intakes is inferred. For example, if one were planning diets for a group of elderly residents in a long-term care facility, it would probably not be appropriate to estimate the distribution of usual intakes from data on a free-living elderly group. The latter group would likely display greater heterogeneity in intakes and thus larger between-person variation in usual intakes than the institutionalized group.

When estimating the distribution of usual intakes, whether from primary or secondary sources, the planner should keep in mind possible sources of error associated with self-reported intakes. Despite corrections to remove the effect of within-person variation, additional random error occurs as a result of errors in dietary assessment methodology, sampling variability, and inaccuracies in nutrient databases. In addition, the underestimation of actual energy intakes is well documented (Johansson et al., 1998; Mertz et al., 1991), and related nutrients may be systematically underestimated as well. Although there is currently no acceptable method to correct for this underestimation, the planner should be aware that such an underestimation of intake could lead to an overestimation of the prevalence of inadequate nutrient intakes, and thus of the actual need for increased intakes to reduce nutrient inadequacy. While the planner is encouraged to plan for adequate nutrients consumed, rather than just adequate nutrients offered or served, the accurate assessment of and subsequent planning for diets as consumed is challenging.

Selecting the Target Prevalence of Inadequacy

In planning diets for groups, the target prevalence of inadequacy is ultimately a matter of judgment. A conservative approach is to aim for a prevalence of 2 to 3 percent. In this case, the likelihood that a randomly selected individual in the group has an inadequate intake would be between 2 and 3 percent, representing a probability of between 0.02 and 0.03. A higher prevalence could be selected, though, and the selected prevalence of inadequacy could vary by nutrient, depending upon available resources.

In setting planning goals for groups, two scenarios are particularly interesting to consider. The first is planning so that the resulting distribution of usual intakes has *all* individuals in the group consuming at least the Recommended Dietary Allowance (RDA), a goal that might appear to be consistent with what practitioners often counsel clients to achieve with their individual diets (Figure 3-2, Panel B). The second is planning such that the median of the target distribution of usual intakes in the group equals the RDA (Figure 3-2, Panel C). This goal appears consistent with current planning applications where individuals in a group are offered foods and meals that provide 100 percent of the RDA. Presumably, this goal reflects the notion that if individuals consume, on average, what is offered, that mean intake will equal the RDA. As shown below, neither of these two scenarios is being proposed or promoted for group planning because each has potentially negative implications.

To examine the implications of these two scenarios, Figure 3-2 compares the target usual nutrient intake distribution for a hypothetical nutrient with an EAR of 50 units, a standard deviation (SD) of requirement of 7.5 units (coefficient of variation [CV] of requirement = 15 percent), and an RDA of 65 units. The intake distribution will simplistically be assumed to be normal, with a standard deviation of usual intake of 18 units. Panel A, with a group prevalence of inadequacy of 2 to 3 percent, is similar to the target usual nutrient intake distribution portrayed in Figure 3-1, while Panels B and C show the two scenarios described above. Several important conclusions are clear from Figure 3-2:

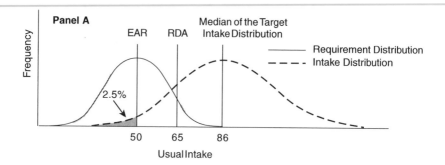

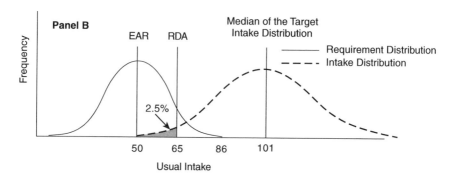

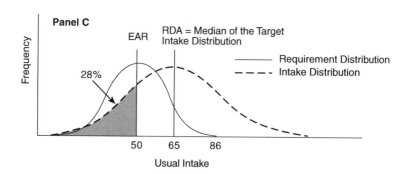

FIGURE 3-2 Panel A: low group prevalence of inadequacy: 2.5 percent of the population has usual intake below the estimated average requirement. Intake distributions are assumed to be normal. Median of the target intake distribution = Estimated Average Requirement (EAR) + 2 Standard Deviations (SD) of *intake* (in this example, the SD of intake = 18 units). Panel B: low individual risk of inadequacy: 2.5 percent of the population has usual intake below the Recommended Dietary Allowance (RDA). Intake distributions are assumed to be normal. Median of the target intake distribution = RDA + 2 SD of *intake* (in this example, SD of intake = 18

- Panel A: planning for a low group prevalence of inadequacy. Around 2 to 3 percent of the group has a usual intake less than the EAR. Approximately 16 percent of the group will have a usual intake less than the RDA for this nutrient with an EAR of 50 units, an SD of requirement of 7.5 units, and an SD of usual intake distribution of 18 units. Note that the median of this target intake distribution is 86 units, considerably higher than the RDA of 65 units.
- Panel B: planning for a low individual risk of inadequacy. Around 2 to 3 percent of individuals have a usual intake less than the RDA. The target usual intake distribution is positioned substantially higher when planning for a risk of inadequacy of no more than 2 to 3 percent for each individual, as opposed to a prevalence of inadequacy of 2 to 3 percent for a group. Only an extremely small proportion of the group is likely to have a usual intake less than the EAR and, thus, the prevalence of inadequacy is essentially zero. Although not shown in the figure, concerns about some individuals exceeding the Tolerable Upper Intake Level may arise when setting a target usual nutrient intake distribution so high.
- Panel C: planning for a target usual nutrient intake with a median equal to the RDA. The target usual nutrient intake distribution (and its median) is substantially lower than for either a low group prevalence of inadequacy or low risk for each individual. Fifty percent of the group will have a usual intake less than the RDA. The prevalence of inadequacy is high. In this example, the proportion of the group with a usual intake less than the EAR is about 28 percent.

The implications of Panel C are extremely important and deserve to be highlighted. When the target usual nutrient intake distribution is positioned to have a median equal to the RDA, the expected prevalence of inadequate intake is fairly high, around 28 percent in this example. The reason for this apparent inconsistency is the variance in usual intake that is observed in most groups. The proportion of the group with inadequate intake when the target usual intake distribution has a median at the RDA is directly proportional to the standard deviation of usual intake. At the extreme, if there were no variance in intake and all individuals in the group con-

---

units). Panel C: higher group and individual risk of inadequacy: target median intake equals the RDA. Intake distributions are assumed to be normal. Median of the target intake distribution = RDA (65 units in this example). EAR = 50 units in this example, with a standard deviation of 7.5 units) and RDA = EAR + 2 SD of *requirement*, or 65 units.

sumed exactly what was offered (100 percent of the RDA), then the prevalence of inadequate intake would be 2 to 3 percent. As a less extreme example, if the standard deviation of usual intake were 9 units rather than the 18 units used above, then the prevalence of inadequacy would be about 15 percent instead of the 28 percent estimated above.

Ultimately planners must decide what is the acceptable prevalence of inadequacy. If planners decide that either a low group prevalence (Panel A) or a low individual risk (Panel B) of inadequacy is the underlying goal, then meals, food plans, and food assistance benefits for groups must offer substantially more than the RDA for the resulting distribution of usual intake to achieve this goal. On the other hand, planners might decide that a target usual nutrient intake distribution with a median intake equal to the RDA is the planning goal (Panel C), assuming that if everyone consumed all that was offered, then the diet would be nutritionally adequate for almost all individuals in the group. However, this is usually not a realistic assumption, and thus the inevitable variation in usual intakes will result in a prevalence of inadequacy that is greater than 2 to 3 percent.

Estimating the Target Usual Nutrient Intake Distribution

As indicated in the previous section, a planner must first determine the acceptable group prevalence of inadequate intakes, whether it is 2 to 3 percent, 28 percent, or any other selected prevalence. Recall that under certain assumptions, the group prevalence of inadequate intakes is simply the proportion of the group with usual intakes less than the EAR. Planning in this case involves positioning the usual intake distribution such that the acceptable group prevalence of inadequate intakes is set at the EAR. This goal is often achieved by examining an existing usual intake distribution and estimating how it would need to change.

Estimating the Target Usual Nutrient Intake Distribution Assuming a Normal Distribution of Usual Intake

To determine the target usual nutrient intake distribution with the selected prevalence of inadequacy, it is useful to examine the admittedly simple example of a normal distribution of usual intake. When it is known that the usual intake distribution approximates normality, as depicted in Figure 3-2, the position of the target usual nutrient intake distribution can be estimated very simply with a table of selected areas under the normal distribution. The median of the target usual intake distribution is the EAR + $Z \times SD_{usual\ intake}$ where Z comes from a table of areas under the curve of a normal distribution. Table 3-1 reproduces part of a table of Z values. For example, as shown in Panel A of Figure 3-2, when the EAR is 50 units and the $SD_{usual\ intake}$ is 18 units, a 2.5 percent prevalence of inadequacy ($Z = 1.96$ at 2.5 percent) would be expected when the median intake was 86 units ($86 = 50 + [1.96 \times 18]$).

Estimating the Target Usual Nutrient Intake Distribution Assuming a Non-Normal Distribution of Usual Intake

In most cases, however, the distribution of usual nutrient intakes is not normally distributed, so the $SD_{usual\ intake}$ cannot be used to identify the position of the target usual nutrient intake distribution. The approach to estimating the target distribution for a non-normal usual intake distribution is similar in principle to the approach described above, although it does not depend on the SD of intakes and a Z value. That is, one first specifies the acceptable prevalence of inadequate intake (such as 2 to 3 percent), and then plans to

TABLE 3-1 Setting the Target Median Intake[a] for Nutrients with Intake Distributions Approximating Normality: Selecting Z Values

Acceptable Group Risk of Inadequate Intakes (%)	Z Value: Multiplier for the Standard Deviation of Intake
0.05	3.27
0.5	2.57
1.0	2.33
1.5	2.17
2.0	2.05
2.5	1.96
3.0	1.88
5.0	1.65
10.0	1.28
15.0	1.03
25.0	0.68
50.0	0.00

[a] Target median intake = EAR + $Z \times SD_{usual\ intake}$, where EAR = Estimated Average Requirement, Z = statistical tool to determine areas under the normal distribution, SD = standard deviation.
SOURCE: Adapted from Steel et al. (1997).

position the usual intake distribution such that the percentile of usual intake associated with this specified prevalence of inadequate intake equals the EAR.

Consider the zinc example presented previously for girls 9 to 13 years of age. Table 3-2 presents descriptive data on the usual intake of zinc for these girls based on data from the Third National Health and Nutrition Examination Survey (NHANES III) as adjusted (IOM, 2001). Recall that the EAR for zinc for girls 9 to 13 years of age is 7 mg, which is approximately equal to the 10th percentile of usual intake. If the planning goal is to have 2 to 3 percent of individuals in a group have usual intake less than the EAR, the distribution of usual intake should be shifted such that the 2nd to 3rd percentile corresponds to 7 mg. That shift is about 0.8 mg, so the target usual nutrient intake distribution would have a median of about 9.4 + 0.8 = 10.2 mg (where 9.4 is the observed median zinc intake for this group), if it is assumed that the shape of the distribution does not change with whatever intervention is required to increase intakes by 0.8 mg.

Note the substantial error that would occur if the distribution of usual intake were assumed to be normal and the median of the target distribution were estimated to be the EAR + 2 × $SD_{usual\ intake}$. In this case, the $SD_{usual\ intake}$ is 3.1 mg and the median of the target distribution would be estimated as 7.0 + (2 × 3.1) = 13.2 mg, which is more than the value of 10.2 mg, as estimated from the non-normal distribution of usual intake.

TABLE 3-2 Distribution of Usual Intake of Zinc, Girls 9 to 13 Years of Age

Percentile of Intake	Zinc Intake (mg)
1st	6.0
2nd	6.1
3rd	6.3
5th	6.5
10th	7.1
25th	8.1
50th	9.4
95th	13.5
99th	15.5

NOTE: Mean intake = 9.6 mg, median intake = 9.4 mg.
SOURCE: Adapted from IOM (2001).

Assuming Stability in the Distribution of Usual Intakes

The methods proposed here for defining the target distribution of usual nutrient intakes for a group all depend on knowledge of the distribution of requirements for the group and an estimate of the shape of the usual nutrient intake distribution within the group. Implicit in these methods is the assumption that the shape of the distribution of usual nutrient intakes is a stable characteristic of the group, and that irrespective of where the desired distribution of usual intakes is positioned, this shape remains unchanged. If intake is normally distributed, this assumption means that the SD of intake remains unchanged. At higher or lower levels of intake, however, it seems likely that the shape of the distribution and the magnitude of the variance in usual intakes may change. Further research is required to determine the nature of such changes.

Precision of the Estimated Prevalence of Inadequate Intakes

An assumption that is fundamental to both dietary planning and dietary assessment is that the EAR cut-point method accurately reflects the group prevalence of nutrient inadequacy. Because the acceptable prevalence of inadequacy is almost always a low number, planners should be aware of the approximate nature of the prevalence estimate. As described elsewhere (IOM, 2000a), the EAR cut-point method appears to be robust in most situations and is therefore a recommended approach. However, the degree of relative error increases when the prevalence of inadequacy is low. Error also arises as a function of the sample size upon which the assessment is based. For example, an estimated prevalence of inadequacy of 3 percent, based on a sample size of 100, could imply a true population prevalence between 0 and 6 percent (95 percent confidence interval). Thus, in practical situations, if one planned for a prevalence of inadequacy of 2 to 3 percent, implemented the plan, assessed the results and found that the prevalence of inadequacy was 5 percent, this should be interpreted as consistent with the planning goal.

Feasibility of Obtaining the Target Usual Nutrient Intake Distribution

The principle underlying the framework for planning for group feeding is that information on the nutrient requirements and usual intakes can be used to develop a plan where intakes will meet the requirements of all but a targeted proportion of the group. In estimating the target usual intake distribution, each nutrient must be considered individually. However, planning diets for groups necessarily requires the development of food plans or menus that will achieve planning goals for the full range of nutrients considered, while at the same time meeting individuals' energy needs. In planning for group feeding, an important question to ask is whether a target usual nutrient intake distribution is attainable (i.e., are adequate resources available).

Recall that the target intake distribution depends on the median nutrient requirement (EAR) and the estimated distribution of usual intakes in the group. If all individuals in a group consume exactly what they are offered in a group-feeding situation, then the SD of intake would be zero and the amount offered would equal the planners' nutrient intake goal. Yet individuals in a group seldom consume exactly what is offered. Some individuals in a group will eat less than what is offered, and in some situations, others may be able to supplement what is offered with foods from other sources.

In general, the feasibility of attaining the target usual nutrient intake distribution depends in part on the variance in usual intakes in the group. Achieving intake targets is easiest in group-feeding situations where the variability in usual intakes is relatively small and relatively stable. In group-feeding situations, such as nursing homes or other long-term care facilities where staff have a good knowledge of food consumption patterns and are able to tailor menu options to meet the preferences of most individuals in the group, target usual nutrient intake distributions may be readily attainable.

Planners may also be able to manipulate the variance in usual intakes to some extent through the design of menus. For example, it may be that offering pizza in a school lunch has an SD of intake considerably smaller than the SD of intake for a less desirable entree. In the former situation, it would obviously be easier to achieve the target usual intake distribution than in the latter, at least for the nutrients provided by pizza.

However, under some circumstances, resource constraints may mean that it is simply not feasible to design diets or meal plans to achieve the target usual intake distribution for a particular nutrient based on a targeted prevalence of inadequacy. In these situations, one alternative may be to consider whether a higher prevalence of inadequacy would be acceptable. Another alternative is to consider program interventions that will attempt to change the shape of the distribution, for example, by targeting the lower tail of the distribution, as discussed later in this chapter. A key advantage of the framework developed here is that it allows planners to estimate the prevalence of inadequacy in advance, thus guiding an evaluation of the feasibility of attaining any selected prevalence level.

Planning for Groups When Assumptions of the EAR Cut-Point Method Are Violated

In the methods presented thus far, the target usual nutrient intake distribution has been set in relation to the EAR as a means to achieve intakes with an acceptably low prevalence of inadequacy. This approach to planning for groups is only appropriate under certain assumptions. These assumptions are:

- the requirement distribution is symmetric;
- the variance of requirements is less than the variance of usual intake; and
- the usual intake of, and requirement for, a nutrient are not correlated.

Alternative approaches to group planning must be employed when any of these assumptions are not met. In most cases, the alternative is based on using the probability approach (NRC, 1986) when planning for group feeding.

What Happens When the Requirement Distribution Is Not Symmetric?

When the distribution of requirements is not symmetric about the median requirement, but instead is positively skewed (e.g., skewed to the right as occurs for iron), the EAR cut-point method *underestimates* the true prevalence of inadequacy in a group (IOM, 2000a). If the requirement is negatively skewed (e.g., skewed to the left), the method *overestimates* the true prevalence. Thus, if planning for normal group feeding involves a nutrient where the requirement distribution is not symmetric, positioning the target usual nutrient intake distribution as a function of the EAR will not achieve the targeted risk of inadequacy. Although little empirical evidence is available on the distribution of requirements for most nutrients, it is often implicitly assumed that the distribution is symmetric around the median requirement.

One nutrient for which it is known that the requirement distribution is not symmetric is iron (IOM, 2001). Thus, the probability approach should be used in planning iron intake for groups.

When the distribution of requirements is skewed, the same principles for normal group feeding apply but the underlying approach used in planning differs. That is, the planning objective remains the same—to position the usual intake distribution such that a specified proportion of the group has a usual intake less than the requirement. Instead of using the EAR cut-point method to define that target usual intake distribution, however, the probability approach can be used. In this case, the first step is to estimate the distribution of usual intakes in the group. The probability approach (NRC, 1986) is then applied to the adjusted distribution of intakes to estimate the prevalence of inadequacy in the group. To determine what level of change in intakes would be required to achieve an acceptably low risk of inadequacy, the distribution of usual intakes is repositioned by adding a constant to each point along the distribution, and the prevalence of inadequacy recalculated. This procedure is repeated, with the estimated usual intake distribution being shifted in increments and the prevalence of inadequacy recalculated until an acceptably low risk of inadequacy is achieved.

For example, use of the probability approach to assess the iron intake of women aged 31 to 50 in the NHANES III survey suggested that 15 to 20 percent of women had inadequate intakes (IOM, 2001). In that survey, median iron intake from food was 12.1 mg/day, and the 5th and 95th percentiles were 7.4 mg/day and 20.3 mg/day, respectively. If the planning goal was to reduce the prevalence of inadequacy to less than 5 percent, iron intake would need to increase. The initial choice of the constant to add to each point in the distribution is arbitrary. In this case, one might begin by adding 1 or 2 mg, and then use the probability approach to estimate the resulting prevalence of inadequacy. If the prevalence was still above the planning goal, additional amounts would be added until assessment using the probability approach indicated that the planning goal had been met.

What Happens When the Variance of Requirements Exceeds the Variance of Usual Intakes?

When the variance of the requirement distribution exceeds the variance in usual intakes in the group, the EAR cut-point method usually results in a biased estimate of the group prevalence of inadequacy. As a result, there will be a bias in estimating the target usual intake distribution that would achieve the targeted prevalence of inadequacy. In this case, the probability approach described above should be used for group planning.

For nutrients for which average requirements have been estimated, the CVs have been assumed to be 10 to 20 percent. Among free-living populations, the between-person variation in usual intakes typically is considerably higher than this, but in institutional settings where residents are fed similar diets (e.g., prison inmates or residents of a long-term care facility), the distribution of usual intakes *may* display less variance than the distribution of individual requirements for a particular nutrient. When this is confirmed or strongly suspected, the probability approach is the preferred method to define the target usual nutrient intake distribution.

What Happens if Usual Intake and Requirement Are Correlated?

Usual intakes for certain nutrients (e.g., energy) increase with higher needs. This results in a situation in which individuals with higher requirements have higher usual intakes, that is, the intake and the requirement for a given individual are correlated rather than independent.

In general, when intake and requirement are correlated, both the EAR cut-point method and the probability approach would overestimate the prevalence of inadequate intake. Thus, the approach presented above of planning for a usual intake distribution when intake and requirement are correlated will overestimate the usual nutrient intake distribution necessary to achieve planning goals.

Can the target usual nutrient intake distribution for food energy be estimated based on either the EAR cut-point method or the probability approach?

No. Empirical evidence suggests a high correlation between usual energy intake and energy expenditure to maintain current body weight. This correlation most likely reflects either the regulation of energy intake to meet needs or the adjustment of energy expenditures to be consistent with usual intake (FAO/WHO/UNU, 1985). Because of this correlation, neither the EAR cut-point method nor the probability approach can be used to assess the proportion of a group with inadequate energy intake and, thus, cannot be used in planning for adequate energy intakes.

What is the expected bias resulting from the correlation between intake and requirement? At correlation levels no larger than 0.25 to 0.30, the bias is likely to be low (see IOM [2000a] for an in-depth discussion). For higher levels of correlation, especially as the correlation between usual intake and requirement approaches 1.0, neither the EAR cut-point method nor the probability approach can be applied to define a target usual intake distribution for group planning.

PLANNING FOR ENERGY AND MACRONUTRIENT INTAKES OF GROUPS

As is true for individuals, the underlying objective of planning for energy intakes of a group is similar to planning for nutrients—to attain an acceptably low prevalence of inadequacy and of potential excess. It should be emphasized that in the context of planning energy intakes for groups, energy requirements are operationally defined as the total energy expenditure required to maintain a group member's current weight and activity level, regardless of whether that weight is desirable. Thus, planned intake represents the amount of energy required to maintain current status, so in this context, "energy requirement" and "total energy expenditure" are used interchangeably.

The approach to planning for energy differs substantially from planning for other nutrients. There are a number of reasons why this is true. For example, because of the serious and pervasive problem of underreporting of energy intakes, estimating the distribution of energy intakes may lead to erroneous conclusions. Second, there is a high correlation of energy intake and total energy expenditure such that neither the probability approach nor the Estimated Average Requirement (EAR) cut-point method can be used. In addition, and of greatest importance, there are adverse effects associated with consuming amounts *above* or *below* the requirement. Thus, instead of determining usual energy intakes to use as a basis for planning, energy expenditure can be estimated based on gender, height, weight, age, and activity levels. By definition, energy expenditure is equal to intake when energy balance exists. Two approaches to meeting this objective could be considered: estimate requirements for the reference person used to establish the Dietary Reference Intakes (DRIs), or obtain an average of estimated requirements for group members.

Estimate Requirements for the Reference Person

At first glance, it might appear reasonable to estimate group energy needs based on the estimated energy requirement (EER) for the reference person used to represent the group when describing the DRIs. For example, if one were planning for a group of low-active men aged 19 to 30, one could estimate the EER for the reference man who was 70 kg in weight and 1.76 m in height who performed a low level of activity, and use this number (about 2,700 kcal) as the target intake for the group. This approach, however, requires that the reference individual represents group average values for age, height, weight, and activity level. For most life stage and gender groups, the reference person weighs less than the average person (e.g., the reference 19- to 30-year-old man weighs 70 kg; the average weight in this age range is 76 kg). Thus, estimating group energy needs based on the reference individual would underestimate group requirements, and the distribution of intakes would not correspond to the distribution of requirements.

Obtain an Average of Estimated Requirements for Group Members

The recommended approach would be to attempt to plan for an average energy intake equal to the average energy expenditure of the group. For example, if one were planning for the energy intake of a group of men aged 19 to 30, one could estimate the energy expenditure for each individual in the group (assuming one had access to data on height, weight, age, and activity level) and then use the average of these values as the average group-planning goal.

Table 3-3 shows an example of how this could be done for a small group of six healthy men. In this hypothetical example, it can be

TABLE 3-3 Example of Estimating an Average Energy Requirement for a Group of Men Aged 19 to 30

Subject	Age (y)	Height (m)	Weight (kg)	Physical Activity Level (physical activity coefficient)	Estimated Energy Requirement[a]
1	21	1.83	95	Sedentary (1.0)	2,961
2	27	1.77	75	Low active (1.11)	2,789
3	25	1.69	60	Active (1.25)	2,757
4	19	1.80	75	Low active (1.12)	2,883
5	30	1.73	80	Very active (1.48)	3,641
6	25	1.75	75	Low active (1.11)	2,796
Total					17,827
Mean					2,971

[a] Energy (kcal) = 661.8 − (9.53 × age [y]) + physical activity coefficient × (15.91 × weight [kg] + 539.6 × height [m]).
SOURCE: IOM (2002).

seen that the average expenditure of the group is 2,971 kcal/day. If 2,971 is used as the average planned intake for this group, it exceeds the estimated requirement of five of the men, and is below the estimated requirement of one large, very active man (in a larger, more homogeneous group, one would expect the estimate to be inadequate for half the men and above the requirement for the other half). However, because intakes and requirements are highly correlated, and assuming that all members of the group have access to food, most members of the group will consume an amount of energy equal to their expenditure. Thus, planning for a mean group intake that approximates the mean estimated requirement should allow a distribution of intakes that corresponds to the distribution of actual requirements.

As with other planning applications, assessing the plan for energy intakes of a group following its implementation would lead to further refinements. In the case of energy, however, assessment would be based on monitoring body weight rather than on reported energy intake (IOM, 2002a).

Planning the Macronutrient Distribution

In addition to planning for a group's mean energy intake, another goal could be to plan for a macronutrient distribution in which the percentages of energy intake of most group members fall within the Acceptable Macronutrient Distribution Ranges that have been recommended for individuals. These ranges exist for total carbohydrate, total fat, n-6 polyunsaturated fatty acids, n-3 polyunsaturated fatty acids, and protein. For adults, the suggested ranges are 45 to 65 percent, 20 to 35 percent, 5 to 10 percent, 0.6 to 1.2 percent, and 10 to 35 percent of energy, respectively (IOM, 2002a).

As an example, consider the distribution of usual intake of energy from protein, carbohydrate, and total fat in women aged 31 to 50 years, shown in Table 3-4, and assume that the planning goal is to have no more than 5 percent below the lower end and no more than 5 percent above the upper end of the acceptable range. For protein, the prevalence of usual intakes both below and above the acceptable range is essentially zero, so one might plan to maintain the current usual intake distribution with a median intake of 15.6 percent of energy.

For carbohydrate, however, approximately 20 percent of women have usual intakes below 45 percent of energy, the lower end of the range. If one uses the approach outlined above to plan for nutri-

TABLE 3-4 Selected Percentiles for Usual Daily Percentage of Total Energy from Protein, Carbohydrate, and Fat for Women Aged 31 to 50 Years, Continuing Survey of Food Intakes by Individuals, 1994–1996, 1998

	AMDR[a] (%)	Percentile								
		1st	5th	10th	25th	50th	75th	90th	95th	99th
Protein	10–35	10.3	11.8	12.5	13.9	15.6	17.4	19.2	20.4	22.7
Carbohydrate	45–65	35.2	40.1	42.6	46.8	51.3	56.0	60.4	63.2	68.9
Fat	20–35	20.2	23.9	25.9	29.3	32.8	36.4	39.6	41.6	45.2

[a] AMDR = Acceptable Macronutrient Distribution Range.
NOTE: Estimates are based on two daily intakes for each respondent in the sample. The Iowa State University (ISU) method was used to estimate individual usual intakes of energy from protein, carbohydrate, fat, and total energy. One gram of protein was assumed to provide 4 kcal of energy, 1 g of carbohydrate was assumed to provide 4 kcal of energy, and 1 g of fat was assumed to provide 9 kcal of energy. A modification of the ISU method was then implemented to estimate the distribution of the nutrient density (Goyeneche et al., 1997).
DATA SOURCE: ARS (1998).
SOURCE: ENVIRON International Corporation and Iowa State University Department of Statistics, as reported in IOM (2002a).

ents and begins by planning to reduce the prevalence of low carbohydrate intakes to 5 percent, one would shift the distribution so that the 5th percentile of intake was 45 percent, or an increase of about 5 percentage points from the observed distribution. The median of that distribution would be 56.3 percent of energy from carbohydrate, compared to the observed 51.3 percent. However, assuming that the shape of the distribution did not change, intake at the 90th percentile would increase to 65.4 percent, such that 10 percent would have carbohydrate intakes above the upper end of the range, rather than the desired 5 percent.

In contrast, for fat the prevalence of intakes below 20 percent of calories is essentially zero (< 1 percent), but over 25 percent of women have usual intakes above the upper end of the range (> 35 percent). To decrease this to 5 percent, one would plan to position the usual intake distribution such that intake at the 95th percentile was 35 percent rather than the observed 42 percent, a decrease of 7 percentage points. The median of that distribution would be 25.8 percent of energy from fat (32.8 − 7 = 25.8). However, assuming the shape of the distribution did not change, the resulting intake distribution would be such that more than 10 percent of women would have intakes below the lower end of the range (23.9 − 7 = 16.9).

One approach to minimizing the proportions of a group that fall below or exceed the acceptable ranges would be to first plan for a low prevalence of inadequate protein intakes (i.e., a low proportion with intakes below the EAR). Because adult women appear to have a low prevalence of inadequacy for total protein, protein intakes could be maintained at the current 15.6 percent of energy, leaving the remaining 84.4 percent of energy to be allocated between fat and carbohydrate. Starting with fat, one might plan for a median intake at the midpoint of the acceptable range, or in this case, about 28 percent of energy. Because macronutrient intakes expressed as a percentage of energy appear to have reasonably symmetrical usual intake distributions (IOM, 2002a), planning for the midpoint would balance the proportions below and above the acceptable range. Finally, the planned median intake of carbohydrate would be determined by difference. In this example, planning for a median intake of 15.6 percent of energy from protein and 28 percent of energy from fat would leave the remaining 56.4 percent to come from carbohydrate. This example does not consider the possible contribution of energy from alcohol. If alcohol is consumed, its energetic contribution should be counted as part of the fat intake (IOM, 2002a). For example, if alcohol contributed 3 percent to energy intake, this amount would be subtracted from the Acceptable Macronutrient Distribution Range for fat, leaving 17 to 32 percent of energy from fat.

The above approach to planning ranges of macronutrient intake, however, might still lead to a situation in which undesirably high proportions of the group have fat or carbohydrate intakes below or above the acceptable range. Accordingly, planners may need to plan an intervention that would change the *shape* of the macronutrient distributions, perhaps focusing on reducing the proportions above the upper boundary of the range for total fat and below the lower boundary of the range for carbohydrate.

PLANNING MENUS TO ACHIEVE TARGET USUAL NUTRIENT INTAKE DISTRIBUTIONS

After the planner has estimated a target usual nutrient intake distribution for each nutrient of interest, this information then needs to be incorporated into a plan of how to feed a group such that the target usual nutrient intake distribution is achieved.

Depending upon the planning context, planning how to achieve this may involve different considerations. As examples, planning may involve developing a menu for a meal to serve at an elderly nutrition center; it may involve determining which foods to offer as a school lunch or as a meal in a prison or other institution; it may mean devising an emergency food ration; or it may require developing a food plan to serve as the basis for a food assistance program or a food guide to use in planning menus for groups.

Regardless of the planning context, planning to achieve the target nutrient intake distribution ultimately involves determining what to offer or serve the individuals in a group. Yet, regardless of what is offered to a group, intakes—the ultimate goal of group planning—will differ from what is offered. Members of the group will vary in what they consume of the foods offered and in the amount of foods that they consume from other sources. Moreover, in most situations, what is offered itself varies. For example, a given menu may offer milk, which may include a choice of whole, reduced fat, skim, or chocolate.

Unfortunately, limited information is available on the link between what is offered and intake, and what information is available most certainly reflects the context in which the planning occurs. Nevertheless, after the planner has estimated a target usual intake distribution for each nutrient of interest, this information needs to be operationalized into a menu or any other instrument (such as food vouchers). Menu planning involves several steps:

1. establishing an initial goal for the nutrient content of the menu that is based on the target usual nutrient intake distribution;
2. determining what foods to offer that will most likely result in a distribution of usual nutrient intake that approximates the target, and thus attains the desired probability of nutrient adequacy; and
3. determining the quantities of foods to purchase, offer, and serve.

Each of these steps is discussed in greater detail below.

Establishing an Initial Goal for the Nutrient Content of the Menu

In a simple situation, where it was assumed that nutrient *intake* equaled the estimated nutrient content of the foods *provided*, and that only a single combination of foods is to be offered, it might appear logical to use the median of the target usual nutrient intake distribution as a goal for the nutrient content of a menu. As described earlier, this would be projected to lead to an intake distribution with the desired prevalence of nutrient adequacy, provided that the shape of the distribution did not change. However, in most group-planning situations, nutrient intakes are less than the estimated nutrient content of the foods provided (i.e., food is not completely consumed). Furthermore, many planning applications involve offering a variety of menu options from which the members of the group will select foods. For these reasons, the planner might aim for a menu that offers a variety of meals with a nutrient content range that includes, or even exceeds, the median of the target usual nutrient intake distribution.

Determining What Foods to Offer

After all the nutrient targets have been set, the planner must select foods that will provide this average level of nutrient *intake* and divide these foods into different meals and snacks. To convert nutrient intake targets into food intakes, planners will usually rely on food guides such as the Food Guide Pyramid, published menus, and previously used menus to design a menu that is likely to result in the target level of adequacy. This will typically be an iterative process, often assisted by nutrient calculation software that allows interactive changes to menus and recalculation of the nutrient levels at each step.

Determining the Quantities of Foods to Purchase, Offer, and Serve

Designing menu *offerings* to meet an *intake* target is a difficult task. Because food selections and food waste vary among groups, and among menus within groups, the appropriate procedures for determining the foods to purchase and offer depend heavily on the particular planning context. Few data are available on the relationship between offerings and intakes, and it is therefore difficult to offer the planner a concrete goal in terms of menu planning when the targets have been determined in terms of nutrient usual intakes. In an attempt to offer practical guidance to planners, several still-to-be-tested assertions may be of use:

- Offering meals with an average nutrient content equal to the median of the target usual nutrient intake distribution is likely to result in lower than planned-for adequacy of intakes. This is because individuals in a group tend to consume less than what is offered to them.
- The relationship between offerings and intakes is likely to be

dependent on context. For example, in planning situations in which individuals' choices are constrained to the offered meal (as in an assisted living facility, perhaps), the intake goals might be easier to achieve than in those cases where individuals get to choose foods from a wide range of options that provide varying levels of specific nutrients (such as in a school cafeteria).

• The shape of the intake distribution is likely to change as menus offered to groups change. Thus, even if the menu offered is designed to achieve the target intake distribution and associated level of nutrient adequacy, it is very important to evaluate the impact of the new menu on intakes, as discussed later in this chapter.

The discussion above clearly highlights the need for more research in this area. As stated, planners must be able to translate the nutrient intake goals into menu offerings, and the knowledge necessary to do so effectively is not available at this time. Experienced planners will draw from their own expertise to construct menus that are more likely to meet nutrient adequacy goals, but research that uncovers the relationship between offerings and intakes in various planning contexts is needed.

Planning Menus for Nutrients with an Adequate Intake

For nutrients where there is insufficient evidence to determine an Estimated Average Requirement, an Adequate Intake (AI) has been established. The AI is expected to maintain a defined nutritional state or criterion of adequacy in essentially all members of a healthy population. The AI has been estimated in a number of different ways (IOM, 1997, 1998a, 2000b, 2001, 2002a). In some cases the AI is based on the observed mean intakes by groups that are maintaining health and nutritional status consistent with meeting requirements. In these cases the AI is similar conceptually to the median of a target usual nutrient intake distribution. In other cases the AI is the level of intake at which subjects in an experimental study met the criterion of adequacy. In these cases the AI is not directly comparable to a target median intake.

Because the derivation of the AI differs substantially among nutrients and among age and gender subgroups, it also is the case that its use in planning group diets varies. The AI can be used as a planning goal as the target median intake of a group if the variability in usual intake of the target population is similar to the variability in intake of the population used to set the AI. However, if the AI is not based on a group median intake of a healthy population, planners must recognize that there is a reduced level of confidence that achieving a median intake at the AI will result in a low prevalence of inadequacy. Furthermore, the AI cannot be used to estimate the proportion of a group with inadequate intakes (IOM, 2000a). Thus, regardless of how the AI has been estimated, it is not possible to use the AI to plan a target distribution of usual intakes with a known prevalence of inadequacy.

Table 3-5 presents a summary of the nutrients for which AIs have been estimated, and notes the cases in which these estimates reflect group mean intakes. The comparability of the target group to the population used to set the AI can be verified by referring to the original DRI reports for the nutrients of interest.

Assessing the Results of Planning

The final step in planning intakes is to assess the effectiveness of the planning process. Such an assessment would follow the recommended procedures for assessing group intakes (IOM, 2000a). There are several reasons why assessment is a crucial component of the framework for group planning. First, planners typically can control only what is offered to individuals in the group, not what they actually eat. Because the goal of planning is to achieve an acceptable group prevalence of inadequacy, then it is clear that to judge the success of the planning activity, intake assessment must occur.

Furthermore, the distribution of intakes that was chosen as the starting point for the planning activity often will not be taken from the group for which intakes are being planned. For example, it may be necessary to start with intake distributions from national surveys. Thus, the planner is making an assumption about the applicability of the distribution to the group of interest.

In addition, a crucial assumption is made when establishing the targets for planning—that shifting the distribution of intakes to a new position does not change the shape of the distribution. If the shape changes, then the estimated target percentiles (including the median) of intake may be incorrect. The shape of the distribution is likely to depend on many factors, including food preferences, the types of foods served, and the amount of food needed to meet each person's energy needs. Thus, there are several reasons to believe the distribution's shape would change if a different selection of foods is served.

Planning group diets is an iterative, ongoing effort in which planners set goals for usual intake, plan menus to achieve these goals,

TABLE 3-5 Nutrients with Adequate Intakes

Nutrient	Life Stage Group	Group Mean Intake
Total fiber	1–18 y	No
	19–50 y	No
	> 50 y	No
	Pregnancy and lactation (all ages)	No
n-6 Polyunsaturated fatty acids	0-12 mo	Yes
	1–18 y	Yes
	19–50 y	Yes
	> 50 y	Yes
	Pregnancy and lactation (all ages)	Yes
n-3 Polyunsaturated fatty acids	0–12 mo	Yes
	1–18 y	Yes
	19–50 y	Yes
	> 50 y	Yes
	Pregnancy and lactation (all ages)	Yes
Calcium	0–12 mo	Yes
	1–18 y	No
	19–50 y	No
	> 50 y	No
	Pregnancy and lactation (all ages)	No
Fluoride	0–12 mo	Yes
	1–18 y	Yes
	19–50 y	Yes
	> 50 y	Yes
	Pregnancy and lactation (all ages)	Yes
Magnesium	0–12 mo	Yes
Phosphorus	0–12 mo	Yes
Selenium	0–12 mo	Yes
Biotin	0–12 mo	Yes
	1–18 y	No
	19–50 y	No
	> 50 y	No
	Pregnancy and lactation (all ages)	No
Choline	0–12 mo	Yes
	1–18 y	No
	19–50 y	No
	> 50 y	No
	Pregnancy and lactation (all ages)	No

continued

TABLE 3-5 Continued

Nutrient	Life Stage Group	Group Mean Intake
Folate	0–12 mo	Yes
Niacin	0–12 mo	Yes
Pantothenic acid	0–12 mo	Yes
	1–18 y	Yes
	19–50 y	Yes
	> 50 y	Yes
	Pregnancy (all ages)	Yes
	Lactation (all ages)	No
Riboflavin	0–12 mo	Yes
Thiamin	0–12 mo	Yes
Vitamin B_6	0–12 mo	Yes
Vitamin B_{12}	0–12 mo	Yes
Vitamin C	0–12 mo	Yes
Vitamin D	0–12 mo	No
	1–18 y	No
	19–50 y	No
	> 50 y	No
	Pregnancy and lactation (all ages)	No
Vitamin E	0–12 mo	Yes
Vitamin A	0–12 mo	Yes
Vitamin K	0–12 mo	Yes
	1–18 y	Yes
	19–50 y	Yes
	> 50 y	Yes
	Pregnancy and lactation (all ages)	Yes
Chromium	0–12 mo	Yes
	1–18 y	Yes
	19–50 y	Yes
	> 50 y	Yes
	Pregnancy and lactation (all ages)	Yes
Copper	0–12 mo	Yes

continued

TABLE 3-5 Continued

Nutrient	Life Stage Group	Group Mean Intake
Iodine	0–12 mo	Yes
Iron	0–6 mo	Yes
Manganese	0–12 mo	Yes
	1–18 y	Yes
	19–50 y	Yes
	> 50 y	Yes
	Pregnancy and lactation (all ages)	Yes
Molybdenum	0–12 mo	Yes
Zinc	0–6 mo	Yes

SOURCE: IOM (2000a, 2002a).

assess whether the planning goals were achieved, and then modify their planning procedures accordingly.

PLANNING INTERVENTIONS TO CHANGE THE SHAPE OF THE INTAKE DISTRIBUTION

In the above approach to group planning, the implicit assumption is that the shape of the usual intake distribution is relatively stable and that planning for group feeding simply involves determining the location of the usual intake distribution. However, many interventions will also alter the shape of this distribution, either intentionally or unintentionally.

Desired changes in the shape of the intake distribution might be to shrink both tails of the distribution or to shrink only the lower or upper tail. Interventions targeted to only those in the lower tail, if successful, would reduce the prevalence of inadequate intakes, while interventions targeted to those in the upper tail would reduce the prevalence of excessive intakes. An intervention to reduce the total variance in usual intakes might reduce the prevalence of both inadequate and excessive intakes. Several types of interventions might be designed to change intake distributions. For example, food fortification programs might select foods that are consumed more by the targeted portion of the group. Nutrition education classes might be held for the proportion of the group particularly at risk of low intakes (perhaps those with less education or those who choose not to eat certain types of foods). Food and nutrition assistance programs target low-income families on the assumption that they are at higher risk of inadequate intakes. Some of these applications are discussed in Chapter 5.

It is not surprising that even perfectly planned interventions may not result in the expected changes in intake. Unfortunately, limited guidance can be offered to planners at this time because detailed examinations of the impact of various types of interventions on the shape of an intake distribution are almost nonexistent. Further research is clearly needed to guide planners when selecting intervention approaches.

4

A Theoretical Approach Using Nutrient Density to Plan Diets for Groups

SUMMARY

In this chapter the use of nutrient densities is proposed as a means to plan diets for groups comprised of distinct subgroups with different nutrient requirements and different usual energy intakes. Two approaches are described. The first relates the median of the target nutrient intake distribution to the mean energy intake of each subgroup within the larger group, for which a diet is being planned. These values are then compared to set a planning goal for the whole group. This approach, however, does not consider the variability of energy intakes within a subgroup, so it may require repeated iterations of planning and assessment. The second approach involves planning for an acceptable nutrient density ratio. This approach takes into account the differences both in energy and nutrient needs of the distinct subgroups to derive target nutrient intake distributions expressed as nutrient densities. The medians of the target nutrient density intake distributions for the various subgroups are then compared to set planning goals for the whole group. Importantly, the methods described here are not designed to plan for desirable body weights (which might require weight loss or gain), but to ensure that nutrients are provided in sufficient concentrations in the diet to satisfy individuals' nutrient needs if they consume sufficient food to maintain energy balance. These approaches are theoretical in nature at this time and should be further explored.

INTRODUCTION

The methods presented in Chapter 3 assume that the planning activity will be conducted for a group of people possessing similar energy and nutrient requirements; for example, girls aged 9 to 13 years or adult men aged 31 to 50 years. Nutrient requirements are specific to life stage and gender, but there are many situations in which planning diets for groups means planning for population groups that include individuals of different genders and ages and thus different nutrient and energy requirements. Planning school meals, for example, typically involves offering meals to both boys and girls of ages ranging from 5 to 18 years. Planning the benefit levels for the U.S. Food Stamp Program must include consideration of the combination of ages and genders present in recipient households. Planning the meals in institutional settings such as prisons or hospitals must recognize differences in residents' requirements related to age, weight, gender, and possibly marked differences in habitual levels of physical activity.

When applying the concept of a target usual intake distribution to planning for groups that include individuals with different energy and nutrient requirements, the heterogeneity of the group must be considered. One approach that has been used is to calculate the average nutrient requirement for individual group members and use this average requirement in planning. The problem with this approach, however, is that even if the planning appears to meet the group need for the nutrient, there is no guarantee that nutrient intakes will be distributed among individuals in the group in a manner to satisfy nutrient requirements. For example, in planning for iron intakes for a group of men and women, simply computing the average iron requirement and planning accordingly does not ensure that individual group members will have their iron requirement satisfied. In fact, when planning diets or menus that provide the average iron requirement, it is likely that food (and iron) will be distributed according to energy needs of the individuals in the group. As a result, there will almost certainly be serious deficits in iron intakes for the women, who have lower energy requirements, and surplus iron intakes for the men with their higher energy requirements (FAO/WHO, 1970). Thus, to achieve a targeted group prevalence of inadequacy, subgroup differences in both nutrient and energy requirements need to be taken into account in the planning process.

The use of nutrient densities has been proposed as one means to account for known differences in the energy and nutrient requirements of specific population subgroups (FAO/WHO, 1970; FAO/ WHO/UNU, 1985; IOM, 1995, 2002b). This approach involves calculating the required nutrient density for the diet such that when individuals' requirements for food energy are achieved, there is a high likelihood that the nutrient requirement for individuals within the group also will be satisfied. In planning for nutrient adequacy, it must be assumed that individuals' usual energy intakes are sufficient for them to maintain energy balance with current levels of physical activity and body energy stores, or in other words, that their energy intake equals their energy expenditure.

Nutrient density is the ratio of the amount of a nutrient in foods to the energy provided by these same foods. Nutrient density is frequently expressed as the amount of the nutrient per 1,000 kcal or MJ of energy.

Although nutrient density may be used to describe foods, meals, diets, or food supplies, its use in dietary planning is primarily to describe daily intake targets.

Using the nutrient density concept, a number of approaches to planning the diets of heterogeneous groups could be considered. The approach used depends in part on whether the intakes being planned will be based on consumption of a single food (e.g., an emergency relief ration) or of varied amounts of multiple foods, the more common planning scenario. A method that can be used to plan for diets consisting of a single food is presented in Appendix C, while two approaches are presented below that could be used to plan intakes when the diet consists of multiple foods.

The first approach to planning using nutrient densities is based on a comparison of the target median nutrient intake to the average energy requirement. This simple approach is based on the methods presented in Chapter 3 and is referred to as the simple nutrient density approach. It involves planning nutrient intakes for the subgroup with the highest median nutrient needs relative to their energy needs (e.g., the most vulnerable subgroup); it is assumed that the other subgroups will obtain adequate nutrient intakes if they fulfill their energy requirements. This approach, while simple and straightforward to implement, does not consider the variability in energy intakes within a subgroup and may therefore result in a prevalence of inadequacy that differs from the planning goal.

The second approach to planning using nutrient densities is based on the distribution of intakes expressed as a nutrient density. Although this approach has not been tested in practical situations, it considers the variability of energy intakes within a subgroup as well as the distribution of nutrient intakes, and therefore offers the most theoretically correct method of determining the appropriate nutrient density to use for planning. It includes examining the distribution of intakes expressed as a nutrient density for each subgroup and determining the target nutrient density distribution for each. The nutrient density to be used for planning should be the highest target nutrient density among the subgroups.

For each of these approaches, an assessment and adjustment of the target distribution as needed should follow the planning activity. For the first approach, which does not consider variability in energy intakes, several iterations of planning and assessment may be needed. The second approach should more accurately identify the correct target nutrient density so fewer assessment iterations would be expected. In addition, each approach should include a comparison of the projected target usual intake distribution to the Tolerable Upper Intake Level (UL) for each subgroup. By planning for a nutrient density that is adequate for the subgroup with the highest needs, it is possible that a substantial proportion of some of the other subgroups will consume diets that exceed the UL.

Each of the methods proposed above requires an estimate of the distribution of usual nutrient intakes in the various subgroups of interest. As described in Chapter 3 and more fully elsewhere (IOM, 2000a), the distribution of usual nutrient intakes for each subgroup can be estimated by assessing the nutrient intakes of a representative sample over at least two nonconsecutive or three consecutive days, and adjusting the observed distribution of nutrient intakes for within-person variation.

An estimate of energy intake is also required. Assuming that the group is in energy balance, one could use estimates of either energy intake or energy expenditure. For the first approach, the *mean* energy intake or expenditure in each subgroup of interest is used, while for the more theoretically correct approach, an estimate of the *distribution* of usual energy intakes or expenditures is needed. As is the case with nutrients, in principle, the distribution of usual energy intakes in each subgroup can be estimated by assessing the energy intakes of a representative sample over two or more days and adjusting the observed distribution of energy intakes for within-person variation. The distribution of energy expenditures in each subgroup can be estimated using the equations developed to estimate the energy expenditure of individuals in the group (IOM, 2002a).

However, both of these estimates (energy intake and energy expenditure) are subject to error. Estimates of energy expenditure obtained using energy expenditure equations require data on height, weight, age, and physical activity level. These estimates may be biased if self-reported values for height and weight are used, as height is frequently overreported and weight underreported, particularly among older adults (Kuczmarski et al., 2001).

Error may also be introduced by assumptions regarding the physical activity level of group members. Because the energy expenditure equations were developed very recently, no data are available on the extent of this error.

On the other hand, as discussed in Chapter 1, problems of systematic underreporting of energy intakes in dietary intake surveys have been documented repeatedly, suggesting that this is likely a widespread problem in intake assessments (Black and Cole, 2001). There is also evidence of systematic overreporting of energy intakes among some individuals (Black and Cole, 2001).

The following discussion assumes that one can approximate the distribution of usual energy intakes in the subgroup of interest by using self-reported energy intake data. It is important to recognize, however, that insofar as systematic reporting errors distort the distribution of usual energy intakes, these errors may seriously bias estimates of the distribution of both nutrient requirements and nutrient intakes expressed as densities. Bias would also exist in estimates of the target median nutrient intake expressed in relation to the mean energy intake. Unfortunately, well-established, validated statistical methods to identify and correct for under- or overreporting energy intakes are currently lacking. Implications of systematic reporting errors on the planning methods presented here are examined at the end of this chapter.

The methods described in this chapter are not designed to plan for desirable body weights (which might require weight gain or loss), but rather to ensure that the nutrients are provided in sufficient concentrations in the individuals' diets to satisfy their nutrient needs if they consume sufficient food to maintain energy balance (e.g., to maintain current body weight).

PLANNING FOR HETEROGENEOUS GROUPS USING A COMPARISON OF TARGET MEDIAN NUTRIENT INTAKE TO MEAN ENERGY INTAKE (OR EXPENDITURE)

The approach presented in this section is an extension of the approach presented in Chapter 3 to plan nutrient intakes of homogeneous groups. It is possible that it may be less accurate than the approach described in the following section that uses the distribution of nutrient intakes expressed as a density; however, because it is less complex to implement, it may serve as an interim approach for planners. Chapter 5 provides specific examples of the two approaches and discusses the differences in results.

Four steps are necessary to derive a target median nutrient intake relative to energy for a heterogeneous group:

1. Obtain the median of the target nutrient intake distribution for each subgroup of interest (as described in Chapter 3).

2. Divide this target median nutrient intake by the mean energy intake or expenditure in each subgroup to obtain the target median nutrient intake relative to energy.

3. Compare the target median nutrient intakes relative to energy for each discrete subgroup to identify the subgroup with the highest nutrient intake required relative to its mean energy intake. Use this to set planning goals for the whole group, but ensure that nutrient intakes of other subgroups will not be above the Tolerable Upper Intake Level.

4. Assess whether the plan was successfully implemented. (This step is particularly important with this approach.)

Step 1. Obtain the target median nutrient intake.

The first step in this approach is to obtain the median of the target nutrient intake distribution for each subgroup, following the approach described in Chapter 3. For nutrients for which an Estimated Average Requirement (EAR) has been determined, the target median nutrient intake is the median of the distribution obtained by repositioning (if necessary) the usual nutrient intake distribution in the subgroup of interest so that an acceptably low proportion of individuals in the subgroup has intakes below the EAR. In the case of iron, for which the requirement distribution is skewed, the probability approach is used in place of the EAR cut-point method in order to estimate the target median nutrient intake.

For nutrients with an Adequate Intake (AI), the AI may be used as a target median nutrient intake. Median intake at the AI should lead to a low prevalence of inadequacy if the AI was set as the median intake of a healthy group and if the variability in usual intake of the group of interest is similar to the variability in intake of the population used to set the AI. When either of these conditions is not satisfied, there will be less confidence that achieving a median intake at the AI will result in a low prevalence of inadequacy.

Step 2. Divide the target median intake by the mean energy intake (or expenditure) for each subgroup of interest.

Once the target median nutrient intake has been identified for each subgroup within the larger group, it is possible to express the nutrient intake in relation to energy, typically per 1,000 kcal. This is done by dividing the target median nutrient intake by the mean energy intake or expenditure. For example, if the target median zinc intake for a group of girls 9 to 13 years of age was 10.1 mg and their mean energy intake was 2,200 kcal, this would represent a target of 4.6 mg/1,000 kcal. This would be done for each subgroup.

Step 3. Identify the subgroup with the reference intake and set planning goals for the entire group.

Once the target median nutrient intakes have been expressed relative to the mean energy intake or expenditure for each subgroup, a decision can be made regarding which subgroup's needs will be used to plan intakes for the entire group. In many cases, one might choose to plan using the needs of the most vulnerable subgroup (e.g., the subgroup with the highest target median nutrient intake relative to mean energy intake or expenditure). Diets that would lead to intakes providing that amount of the nutrient per 1,000 kcal would then be planned (e.g., for zinc, if the vulnerable subgroup was girls 9 to 13 years of age, the goal for intake would be 4.6 mg of zinc/1,000 kcal). If the needs of this subgroup are met, the needs of other subgroups should be satisfied and the group prevalence of inadequacy should be low. Alternatively, if the needs of the most vulnerable subgroup would lead to intakes by other subgroups that are excessive (and perhaps above the UL), it may be preferable to use a less vulnerable subgroup to plan for the group as a whole and to target the most vulnerable subgroup using education programs, special foods, or targeted supplementation.

Step 4. Assess whether the plan was successfully implemented.

Assessing the adequacy of the group's nutrient intakes is particularly critical when this approach to dietary planning is used. By using only the mean energy intake or requirement of each subgroup, it fails to consider the variability of energy intakes among members of a subgroup. Accordingly, those with very low energy intakes may not meet their nutrient requirements. Planners using this approach must be willing to alternate planning and assessment until the goals are achieved because the actual prevalence of inadequacy that results from this approach may be quite different from the level that was the target.

PLANNING FOR HETEROGENEOUS GROUPS USING THE DISTRIBUTION OF NUTRIENT INTAKES EXPRESSED AS A DENSITY

This section describes an approach to establish a target nutrient density intake distribution for each of the subgroups in a heterogeneous group, assuming multiple foods with different densities are consumed. It could also be used to plan for a group consisting of a single life stage and gender. The first step in the procedure is as described in Chapter 3: obtain a target usual nutrient intake distribution in each of the subgroups so that an acceptably low proportion of individuals in each subgroup have an inadequate intake of the nutrient. The target distribution of usual intakes expressed as nutrient densities in each of the subgroups is derived relative to the distribution of nutrient and energy requirements in each of the subgroups directly, and provides the planning goal for each subgroup.

Three steps are necessary to derive a target usual density intake distribution.

1. Obtain the target distribution of usual nutrient intakes for each subgroup of interest.

2. Combine the target distribution of usual nutrient intakes with the usual energy intake (or expenditure) distribution in each subgroup to obtain the target distribution of usual nutrient intakes expressed as densities.

3. Compare the estimated target median density intake for each discrete subgroup to identify the reference nutrient density and set planning goals for the whole group, but ensure that nutrient intakes by other subgroups do not exceed the Tolerable Upper Intake Level (UL).

Step 1. Obtain the target distribution of usual nutrient intake.

The first step in planning intakes for a heterogeneous group is to obtain the target usual nutrient intake distributions for each subgroup, following the approach described in Chapter 3. For nutrients for which an Estimated Average Requirement (EAR) has been determined, the target usual nutrient intake distribution is obtained by repositioning (if necessary) the usual nutrient intake distribution in the subgroup so that an acceptably low proportion of individuals in the subgroup have intakes below the EAR. In the case of iron, for which the requirements distribution is skewed, the probability approach is used in place of the EAR cut-point method in order to estimate the position of the target usual nutrient intake distribution.

In Chapter 3 and in the simple approach described in the previous section in this chapter, the planning tool of interest was the *median* of the target usual intake distribution. Here, however, the entire *target usual nutrient intake distribution* is of interest. In order to establish a target nutrient density intake distribution, it is necessary to account for the variability in nutrient and energy intakes among individuals. If the goal is to plan intakes when each of the subgroups is provided a separate diet (as would be the case, for example, in an institution that houses men, women, and young individuals separately), then the planner needs to proceed no further. The methods presented in Chapter 3, and briefly revisited here, suffice to plan intakes for a subgroup that is homogeneous with respect to age and gender. However, if a single diet will be provided to a larger group composed of individuals from the various subgroups, then the planner needs to account for the differences in energy consumption among individuals in different life stage and gender groups.

Step 2. Obtain the target nutrient density intake distributions.

Once the target usual nutrient intake distribution for each life stage and gender subgroup of the larger group has been established (Step 1), it is possible to determine the target usual intake distribution of the nutrient expressed as a density. The target distribution of usual intakes estimated in terms of nutrient densities will be such that an acceptably low proportion of individuals in each subgroup (in the example, 2 to 3 percent) have inadequate nutrient intakes.

While the method presented in Chapter 3 essentially consisted of repositioning the usual nutrient intake distribution, an additional step is needed when planning for a heterogeneous group. The target usual nutrient intake distribution must be combined with the distribution of usual energy intakes in each subgroup to obtain the target nutrient density intake distribution. The difference here is that while the objective is to obtain a target intake distribution for the nutrient expressed as a density, the density intake distribution cannot be directly compared to the nutrient requirement distribution to determine how it should be repositioned. Thus it is necessary to add an intermediate step to the procedure which consists of deriving first the target usual nutrient intake distribution for each subgroup, as was described in Step 1 above. The steps necessary to carry out this derivation are explained in detail below.

Recall that nutrient density intake is defined as the units of a nutrient consumed per 1,000 kcal. Thus, if an individual consumes 2,000 kcal and 104 mg of vitamin C, then that individual consumes a diet with a vitamin C density of 52 mg/1,000 kcal. Therefore, if one knows an individual's usual nutrient intake and her or his usual energy intake, it is possible to calculate the nutrient density intake for that individual. The calculation above can be taken one step further if one considers a group in which individuals vary in their usual nutrient intake. In the unlikely case in which everyone in the group has the exact same usual energy intakes, say 2,000 kcal, then given the distribution of usual nutrient intakes in the group, it is a simple matter to calculate the usual intake distribution of the nutrient expressed as a density: simply divide each usual nutrient intake in the group by 2,000 and multiply by 1,000. However, individuals vary in the amount of energy they consume, and therefore the derivation of the *distribution* of usual intakes of the nutrient expressed as a density given the usual nutrient and energy intake distributions is a bit more challenging. In this more realistic scenario, it is necessary to take into account that individuals vary not only on the amount of the nutrient they consume, but also on the amount of energy they consume.

Suppose that an individual from the subgroup has a vitamin C intake of 70 mg. If it is assumed that the correlation between vitamin C intake and energy intake is moderate to low, then that nutrient intake level may correspond to different combinations of energy intakes and thus vitamin C intakes per 1,000 kcal. For example, the usual intake of 70 mg may result in a vitamin C density intake of 46.7 mg/1,000 kcal if the individual consumes 1,500 kcal/day or in a density intake of 31.8 mg/1,000 kcal if the individual's energy consumption is 2,200 kcal/day.

The simple example above illustrates the importance of accounting for the variability in usual energy intakes among individuals in the subgroups that comprise the larger group. Given each possible usual nutrient intake in the subgroup, one must calculate each of the nutrient density intakes that may result given the distribution of energy intakes in the same subgroup. To account for the variability in energy intakes among individuals in the subgroup, average the nutrient density intakes over the distribution of energy intakes in the subgroup. The average is weighted by the frequency of consumption of each energy level in the group. To obtain this average density intake corresponding to each nutrient intake in the subgroup, the following calculation is used:

$$\text{Average nutrient density intake} = (1/\Sigma_j \text{ frequency}_j) \, \Sigma_{j=1}^{n} \, (\text{usual} \\ \text{nutrient intake/usual energy intake}_j) \times \text{frequency}_j \times 1{,}000 \quad (1)$$

where n denotes the number of energy intake levels in the subgroup, and the subscript j indicates that for each nutrient intake in the subgroup, the summation above must be carried out for each energy intake level. The weights in the summation above are given by the frequencies of consumption of each energy level. For example, in a group of women aged 19 to 50 years, consumption of energy below 500 kcal or above 8,000 kcal would be associated with low frequencies, whereas energy consumption of around 1,500 to 3,000 kcal would be observed more frequently. The calculation above is carried out for each nutrient intake level in the subgroup. As a result, a distribution of density intakes is obtained in the subgroup by combining a target nutrient intake distribution and an actual (unchanged) usual energy intake distribution.

To illustrate this, consider a hypothetical group of 25 men. Intake data were collected from each of these men on two nonconsecutive days, and the intakes were adjusted to estimate usual intake of nutrient Y and usual intake of energy. This group is very unusual, as its nutrient intake distribution at baseline is flat: five men each have usual intakes of 8 units, 9 units, 10 units, 11 units, and 12 units of nutrient Y. The group's energy intake distribution is also unusual: five men each have intakes of 2,000, 2,200, 2,300, 2,500, and 3,000 kcal. Further, these energy intakes are distributed so that each nutrient intake level is represented by all five energy intakes.

The EAR for nutrient Y is 10 units, so at baseline, 10 of the men have usual intakes below the EAR. In this scenario, the planning goal is to have a prevalence of inadequacy that is essentially zero. Accordingly, the target usual nutrient intake distribution is obtained by shifting the baseline distribution up by 2 units, leading to usual intakes of 10, 11, 12, 13, and 14 units of nutrient Y for the men.

To derive the target usual nutrient *density* distribution, each value in the target nutrient intake distribution is paired with each value from the energy intake distribution, as shown in Table 4-1. As shown in the fourth column of the table, the target nutrient density intake distribution ranges from 3.33 units/1,000 kcal to 7.0 units/1,000

TABLE 4-1 Deriving a Target Nutrient Density Distribution for a Hypothetical Group of 25 Individuals

Usual Nutrient Intake Distribution (units of nutrient Y)	Usual Energy Intake Distribution (kcal)	Target Nutrient Intake Distribution (units of nutrient Y)	Target Nutrient Density Intake Distribution (units/ 1,000 kcal)	Intake Resulting from Meals with Average Density
8	2,000	10	5.0	10.18
8	2,200	10	4.55	11.20
8	2,300	10	4.35	11.71
8	2,500	10	4.0	12.72
8	3,000	10	3.33	15.27
9	2,000	11	5.5	10.18
9	2,200	11	5.0	11.20
9	2,300	11	4.78	11.71
9	2,500	11	4.4	12.72
9	3,000	11	3.67	15.27
10	2,000	12	6.0	10.18
10	2,200	12	5.45	11.20
10	2,300	12	5.22	11.71
10	2,500	12	4.8	12.72
10	3,000	12	4.0	15.27
11	2,000	13	6.5	10.18
11	2,200	13	5.91	11.20
11	2,300	13	5.65	11.71
11	2,500	13	5.2	12.72
11	3,000	13	4.33	15.27
12	2,000	14	7.0	10.18
12	2,200	14	6.36	11.20
12	2,300	14	6.09	11.71
12	2,500	14	5.6	12.72
12	3,000	14	4.67	15.27
Average			5.09	

kcal, and has an average of 5.09 units/1,000 kcal. The intakes that would result from meals planned to contain this density of nutrient Y are shown in the fifth column of Table 4.1. It can be seen that none of the men would have intakes below the EAR of 10 units, so the planned-for very low prevalence of inadequacy would be attained.

In practice, it is not really necessary to proceed with the average over all energy consumption levels as above, nor is it necessary to know the frequency of consumption associated with each energy level. The average above can be more easily calculated using a sampling, or Monte Carlo, approach as follows: first, for each usual nutrient intake, randomly select a number m of usual energy intakes from the distribution of energy intakes, and second, compute the following quantity:

$$\text{Average nutrient density intake} = (1/m) \sum_{j=1}^{m} (\text{usual nutrient intake}/\text{energy intake}_j) \times 1{,}000 \qquad (2)$$

Here, m is typically much smaller than n, so that the sum in expression (2) is less computationally demanding than that shown in expression (1). As a guideline, in the example presented in Chapter 5, the value of n for women is approximately 4,500, but only 400 randomly selected energy consumption levels were drawn from the usual energy intake distribution in the group in order to compute the approximation in (2). In fact, a value of m as low as 50 or 100 would have provided a good approximation to the average given in (1). If the m energy intakes are drawn at random from the distribution of usual energy intakes in the subgroup, then the average in (2) is self-weighting. This is because energy intake levels will be drawn more or less frequently depending on the probability associated with each energy intake level in the usual energy intake distribution. That is why the frequency associated with each level of energy consumption does not appear in equation (2).

Either one of the two calculations presented above would produce an average (over the individual's likely levels of energy consumption) nutrient density intake. To simplify the calculations even further, the weighted average above does not have to be computed for each nutrient intake level in the subgroup in order to obtain an approximation of the density intake distribution of the subgroup. Just like in the case of the Monte Carlo average, it is possible to draw at random a number q, also typically smaller than n, of usual nutrient intakes from the target usual nutrient intake distribution in the subgroup. The average (over the range of likely levels of energy consumption) density for each of the q usual nutrient intakes drawn from the distribution in the subgroup would then be calculated as indicated in either of the two expressions presented above. In the example in Chapter 5, $q = 400$, so that about 10 percent of the usual vitamin C intakes for women were drawn from the target usual intake distribution to compute the individual weighted averages using equation (2). Except in the unlikely event in which the correlation between usual nutrient intakes and usual energy intakes is high, the numerical approach detailed in either expression (1) or (2) will produce a usable approximation of the distribution of target nutrient density intakes for a group.

Step 3. Identify the reference nutrient density distribution and set planning goals for the whole group.

Once the target nutrient density distributions have been defined for each distinct subgroup in the population of interest, it is recommended that the distribution with the highest median nutrient density intake among the subgroups be considered the reference nutrient density distribution for the population for planning purposes.

For the subgroup with the highest target median nutrient density, the planned diet should achieve the targeted prevalence of inadequacy. For all other subgroups, the prevalence of inadequacy will be even lower since the nutrient density of the planned diet will exceed their needs. Thus for the population as a whole, the risk of inadequacy will be lower than the level set for the subgroup with the highest target nutrient density.

The target nutrient density intake distribution is obtained from an adequate target nutrient intake distribution, and therefore the resulting target distribution of nutrient density intakes meets the criterion for adequacy that was selected. It is also important to monitor the proportion of individuals whose intakes of the nutrient might exceed the UL.

For some nutrients (notably iron), prioritization of the needs of the subgroup with the highest requirement relative to energy can result in the selection of a target median nutrient density that far exceeds the needs of all other subgroups. Under these circumstances, planners must consider the risk that members of subgroups with lower nutrient requirements relative to energy may achieve intake levels in excess of the UL. They must also consider the cost-effectiveness of providing such a nutrient-dense diet for all subgroups. Under some circumstances, it might be deemed more appropriate to select a lower target nutrient density for the group as a whole and employ direct interventions for the one or two population subgroups in which the prevalence of inadequacy would be above the desired level. This should not be seen as a weakness of the nutrient density approach. Rather, this approach enables the identification of such planning issues.

The strength of the nutrient density approach to planning for groups comprised of individuals from different life stage and gender groups is that the method enables planners to systematically take into account both the specific nutrient requirements of various subgroups and their differing energy needs. The effectiveness of this approach hinges on the ability to implement it and on the validity of the assumptions that underpin it.

TECHNICAL CONSIDERATIONS OF THE NUTRIENT DENSITY DISTRIBUTION APPROACH

Although the nutrient density distribution approach described above is a promising tool for planning group diets, several important issues must be considered.

Nutrients for Which an Adequate Intake Has Been Established

The nutrient density distribution approach to planning group diets cannot be used for nutrients with an Adequate Intake (AI). The reference nutrient density ratio links the requirement distribution of the nutrient and the usual intake distribution of the nutrient to obtain a target nutrient intake distribution (as described in Chapter 3), and then expresses this distribution as a density. Thus, this approach cannot be used in planning for nutrients with AIs because in these cases there is no knowledge of the requirement distribution of the nutrient. Although the simple approach using the median nutrient density presented in the previous section can be used for nutrients with an AI, planners need to be aware of the limitations of this method.

Correlation Between Nutrient Intakes and Energy Intakes

A premise of the nutrient density distribution approach to planning intakes of heterogeneous groups is that the correlation between usual nutrient intakes and usual energy intakes is moderate to low. This assumption permits computing the simple Monte Carlo average that results in a target distribution of nutrient density intakes in each subgroup. The low correlation assumption may not hold since it would be expected that, in general, higher energy consumption would imply higher intake of the nutrient. However, as discussed above, planning intakes for a group in terms of densities would most often imply a change in the relationship between energy and nutrient consumption, one objective being to provide more units of the nutrient per 1,000 kcal of energy in the diet. If, however, assuming low correlation between nutrient and energy intake is deemed unrealistic, in principle their relationship could be modeled, and the Monte Carlo average presented in equation (2) above could be improved. Otherwise, the target density intake distribution in each subgroup could be derived directly from the target *joint* intake distribution of the nutrient and energy. In the latter case, the methods presented in Chapter 3 for a single nutrient would need to be extended accordingly to address the problem of estimating the target intake distribution of two nutrients jointly (one of them being energy). A simplified first approximation of the density approach to planning intakes for heterogeneous groups is presented here, on the assumption that the correlation between energy and nutrient intakes may not be so high as to significantly affect the derivation of the target median nutrient density for the group. However, more research is needed to explore the full implications of this assumption.

The Impact of Reporting Errors

As noted previously, there is ample evidence to suggest that underreporting is a serious problem in dietary intake surveys. The use of doubly labeled water methods to determine energy expenditure has facilitated identification of underreporting in energy intakes, but it is unclear how the reporting of other nutrients is affected by this phenomenon. At present, well-established, validated methods are lacking to identify and correct for systematic reporting errors in individual intakes. Thus it is impossible to determine the impact of underreporting on the planning methods proposed here. Nonetheless, the sources and probable direction of errors associated with underreporting are explored below, considering the particular ways in which self-reported intake data are used in the proposed application of the distribution of nutrient densities to plan for heterogeneous groups. Note that while the discussion below relates primarily to the nutrient density distribution approach, the issues raised are equally relevant to the simple approach that relies on the estimated median energy intake.

The estimated distribution of usual energy intakes is required to derive a distribution of nutrient requirements expressed as densities when planning intakes of a single food or of a diet composed of a variety of foods with similar nutrient density. In planning for heterogeneous groups under normal circumstances (e.g., where individuals consume diets that comprise multiple foods with varying nutrient densities), both nutrient and energy intake data are required. The estimated distribution of usual nutrient intakes is required to estimate the target nutrient intake distribution (see Chapter 3). The estimated distribution of usual energy intakes is necessary to express the target usual nutrient intake distribution in terms of target nutrient densities. Underreporting may bias both the nutrient and energy intake distributions.

The impact of underreporting on estimates of target usual intake distributions expressed as nutrient densities is likely to vary depending on the nutrient of interest. If some of the energy intakes are systematically underreported, but the target nutrient intake distribution is less affected by underreporting, then some overestimation of nutrient requirements in relation to energy would occur. If energy and nutrient intakes have both been underreported to the same extent, then the target density intake distribution may be less biased. However, this assumption of "proportional underreporting" is probably not valid. A more likely scenario is that intakes of energy and the nutrient in question have been disproportionately underreported. The distribution of target usual nutrient intakes expressed as densities will then also be estimated with error, but the nature and magnitude of the error is unknown. The extent of this problem would depend on the number of underreported intakes, the extent of underreporting in energy versus nutrient intakes, and the magnitude of underreporting in the intake data used.

One way to avoid the potential for systematic errors in self-reported energy intakes to skew the distribution of nutrient density requirements might be to approximate the distribution of usual energy intakes from the distribution of energy requirements in the group. Given the high correlation between individuals' energy intakes and energy expenditure, usual energy intake should equal energy expenditure if individuals are in energy balance. Thus, the distribution of usual energy intakes could be constructed by estimating the distribution of energy requirements for the subgroup. Equations to predict energy requirements are provided for individuals with a body mass index (BMI) of > 18.5 and < 25 (IOM, 2002a). Another set of equations is provided to predict total energy expenditure for individuals with BMI ≥ 25. Application of these equations requires knowledge of each individual's age, sex, height, and weight, and sufficient information to classify the individual into one of four broad categories of physical activity levels. In applying the equations to estimate the distribution of usual energy intakes, it is also necessary to take into account the variation in requirements of individuals, estimated by the standard deviation of the prediction.

While this approach provides an alternative to the use of self-reported intake data, it also has some serious limitations. The accuracy of the energy expenditure estimates hinges on the applicability of the equations (and their variance estimates) for the particular group of interest and on the accuracy of the available data on an individual's height, weight, and physical activity level. All of these parameters are subject to measurement error, particularly if self-reported data are used. Furthermore, use of the energy expenditure equations does not eliminate the need to use self-reported nutrient intake data to obtain an estimate of the target nutrient intake distribution.

The use of self-reported dietary intake data is likely to be unavoidable in planning for groups. Clearly, more research is needed to enable planners to identify the nature and magnitude of systematic reporting errors in these data and to statistically adjust planning applications when such errors are present.

An algorithm for the group planning applications presented here and in Chapter 3 is summarized in Figure 4-1. It should be noted, however, that the approaches described are largely theoretical at this stage. More research is required to address specific technical issues, test the effectiveness of the proposed approaches in "real-life" settings, and refine their practical application.

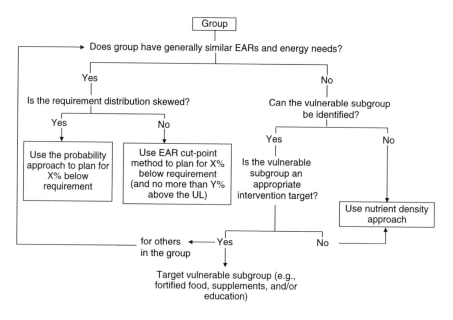

FIGURE 4-1 Schematic decision tree for planning group diets.

5

Examples of Planning for Groups

SUMMARY

Several applications of group planning are presented in this chapter. Two examples focus on normal group feeding situations where the distribution of intakes is shifted but the shape of the distribution is not explicitly changed. Two examples focus on planning for heterogeneous groups using a simple and a complex (but theoretically more correct) nutrient density approach. The final two examples discuss the problem of planning interventions designed to change the shape of the usual intake distribution of one or more nutrients in a targeted population group.

It is often difficult to plan diets that will achieve exactly the desired effect. Therefore, when planning normal diets or dietary interventions it is critically important to assess the likely effects not only on the target group, but also on other groups that would be affected by the intervention.

Important unpredictable factors such as food preferences, participation rates in food assistance programs, or population-based educational programs make the job of an intervention planner very difficult. Typically, forecasting the effect of an intervention is not straightforward, and several cycles of planning followed by assessment may be needed. The applications developed in this chapter are hypothetical.

INTRODUCTION

Planning diets for population subgroups is carried out in many diverse settings and thus has multiple and varied applications. Some of the more visible group-planning applications include planning diets for institutionalized groups, food and nutrition assistance programs, food fortification, nutrition education for groups, and military food and nutrition planning.

The discussion below provides an in-depth analysis of six specific planning applications. Examples (1) an assisted living facility for seniors and (2) school nutrition programs, present the principles described in Chapter 3 for shifting the distribution of usual intakes. Examples (3) a group of teen boys, adult men, and adult women using the simple nutrient density approach and (4) a group of teen boys, adult men, and adult women using the nutrient density distribution approach, present the approaches described in Chapter 4. Finally, examples (5) nutrient supplementation and (6) food fortification, illustrate how interventions intended to shift the distribution of usual intakes may also change the *shape* of the usual intake distribution. This discussion is not intended to prescribe how these planning activities should be conducted. Rather, based on the principles for group planning developed in Chapters 3 and 4, the discussion of these examples is intended to present the issues involved in these planning applications.

The group-planning framework should be applied in pilot situations before it is adopted for large-scale programs.

PLANNING DIETS IN AN ASSISTED-LIVING FACILITY FOR SENIOR CITIZENS

An example of planning diets for institutionalized groups is menu planning for senior citizens who reside in an assisted-living facility. Menus planned for these institutions usually assume that the residents have no other sources of foods or nutrients, and thus the menus are designed to meet all nutrient needs of the residents.

Based on the framework developed in Chapter 3, the goal of menu planning is to provide meals that supply adequate nutrients for a high proportion of the residents, or conversely, to ensure that the prevalence of inadequate intakes are acceptably low among the residents. An important note, and caveat perhaps, is that to fully implement the planning approaches described in this report, data on usual intakes must be available. Unfortunately, such data are seldom available; planners for these and other institutionalized groups (e.g., prisons, boarding schools) frequently do not collect dietary intake data in order to evaluate their menu planning. It is possible to generate usual intake data on the target population through daily food intake records or intake recalls on each individual. However, if the facility is large (e.g., more than 100 residents), intakes could be measured on a representative subsample of residents. Using this technique, two nonconsecutive days or three consecutive days of food intake records or recalls are necessary. Alternatively, records of amounts served and plate waste data for individuals monitored, again for a minimum of two nonconsecutive or three consecutive days, can be used. In both cases, data should be adjusted to remove within-person variability and to obtain the usual nutrient intake distribution by using procedures such as those developed by Nusser and colleagues (1996) or the National Research Council (NRC, 1986).

Another possibility is to use usual nutrient intake distributions from another group in which the members are of similar age to the target group. Ideally, such data would also be for a similar (e.g., gender mix, ethnicity) institutionalized population, since the variation in the distribution of usual intakes is likely to differ among individuals who live in institutionalized settings and those who do not. If such comparable usual intake data are not available, then the only option may be to use usual intake distributions from national surveys such as the Continuing Survey of Food Intakes by Individuals (CSFII) or the Third National Health and Nutrition Examination Survey (NHANES III).

From the most appropriate data set available as described above, the planner examines the proportion of the group with usual intakes less than the Estimated Average Requirement (EAR) (for each of the nutrients for which EARs have been established) as an estimate of the prevalence of inadequate intakes. If the prevalence is unacceptably high for one or more nutrients, then intakes need to be increased. As described in Chapter 3, to estimate the amount of the increase for a given nutrient, the difference between the EAR for that nutrient and the usual intake level corresponding to the selected percentile of the current usual intake distribution (which is the chosen acceptable prevalence of inadequacy) is determined. The median usual intake should be increased by this amount, assuming the shape of the distribution is not expected to change. It is crucial to reassess intakes after the change is made, especially if the change is large, because it is possible (even likely) that the shape of the distribution will change.

As an example, consider a planner who is developing a menu for an assisted-living facility in which the residents are retired nuns aged 70 years and above. For this age group, the EAR for vitamin B_6 is 1.3 mg/day (IOM, 1998a). Assume that no data can be located on the distribution of usual intakes of this group or a similar group, and that resources are not available to conduct a dietary survey in the institution. How could the planner proceed to determine the target intake distribution of vitamin B_6 needed to attain an acceptable prevalence of inadequacy?

Step 1. Determine an acceptably low prevalence of inadequacy.

For vitamin B_6, the EAR was set at a level adequate to maintain plasma pyridoxal phosphate levels at 20 nmol/L (IOM, 1998a). This plasma level is not accompanied by observable health risks, and thus allows a moderate safety margin to protect against the development of signs or symptoms of deficiency. This cutoff level was selected recognizing that "its use may overestimate the B_6 requirement for health maintenance of more than half the group" (IOM, 1998a). For this reason, assume that the planner has determined that a 10 percent prevalence of inadequacy (i.e., 10 percent with intakes below the EAR) would be an acceptable planning goal.

Step 2. Determine the target usual nutrient intake distribution.

Next, the planner needs to position the intake distribution so the nutrient intake goals are met. In this example, the planner decides that the prevalence of inadequacy in the group will be set at 10 percent, and as a result the usual intake distribution of the group should be positioned such that only 10 percent of the group has usual intakes less than the EAR. Using the EAR as a cut point for estimating the prevalence of inadequate intakes builds directly on the approaches previously described for assessing intakes (IOM, 2000a).

Because data on the usual nutrient intake distributions of the residents are not available, other sources must be used to estimate the target usual nutrient intake distribution. Data on the distribution of usual dietary intakes of vitamin B_6 from CSFII (conducted in 1995), NHANES III (conducted between 1988 and 1994), and the Boston Nutritional Status Survey (conducted between 1981 and 1984) are available (IOM, 1998a).[1] The adjusted percentiles for

---

[1] Caution should be used when selecting data sets. If more recent data sets were used in this example, it would provide a better reflection of changes in fortification levels.

women aged 70 years and above (in the Boston survey, aged 60 years and above) are summarized in Table 5-1. Assuming there are no changes in the shape of the distribution, the amount of the shift can be calculated as the additional amount of the nutrient that must be consumed to reduce the proportion of the group that is below the EAR. This is accomplished by determining the difference between the EAR and the intake at the acceptable prevalence of inadequacy (in this case, the 10th percentile of the usual intake distribution). Examination of the data from the three surveys shows that estimated usual intakes of vitamin B_6 vary by as much as 30 percent among the surveys. As a result, the difference between the EAR of 1.3 mg and the intake at the 10th percentile varies, depending on which data are used: for NHANES III the difference is 0.26 mg (1.3 mg – 1.04 mg = 0.26 mg); for CSFII, the difference is 0.42 mg (1.3 mg – 0.88 mg = 0.42 mg), and for the Boston survey, the difference is 0.7 mg (1.3 mg – 0.6 mg = 0.7 mg). In this example, the planner may have no reason to choose data from one particular survey as "more applicable" to his group than another, so he may estimate target usual nutrient intake distributions using all three data sets. Accordingly, the target intake distributions shift up by 0.26 mg, by 0.42 mg, and by 0.7 mg using NHANES III, CSFII, and the Boston survey, respectively. In each case the target usual nutrient intake distribution would lead to the accepted prevalence of inadequacy. Rather than choosing one set of survey data over another, the planner could simply average the summary measures described in the next section.

TABLE 5-1 Selected Percentiles of the Distributions of Usual Intake of Vitamin B_6 from Foods in Older Women

Study[a]	n	Percentile of Usual Intake Distribution of Vitamin B_6 (mg/day)						
		5th	10th	25th	50th	75th	90th	95th
CSFII	221	0.76	0.88	1.11	1.41	1.76	2.12	2.35
NHANES III	1,368	0.92	1.04	1.24	1.53	1.93	2.43	2.76
Boston	281	0.5	0.6	0.7	1.0	1.3	1.6	1.8

[a] CSFII = Continuing Survey of Food Intakes by Individuals (women > 70 y), NHANES III = Third National Health and Nutrition Examination Survey (women > 70 y), Boston = Boston Diet Study (women > 60 y).
SOURCE: IOM (1998a).

Step 3. Select a summary measure of the target usual nutrient intake distribution to use in planning.

After the planner has estimated a target usual intake distribution, this information needs to be operationalized into a menu. In order to do this, the planner will first have to select a summary measure of the target usual nutrient intake distribution to use as a tool in planning the menu. The median of the target intake distribution is the most useful; it can be calculated as the median of the current intake distribution, plus (or minus) the amount that the distribution needs to shift to make it the target usual intake distribution.

In the current example, although the baseline intakes at the 10th percentile and the median differ among the three surveys, the estimates of the medians of the target usual intake distributions are quite similar, as shown in Table 5-2. Assuming that a 10 percent prevalence of intakes below the EAR was considered acceptable, a median intake for vitamin B_6 of 1.7 to 1.8 mg/day would be the planning goal. Accordingly, the menu would need to be planned so that vitamin B_6 intakes would be at this level.

Estimates of target nutrient intakes must be converted to estimates of foods to purchase, offer, and serve that will result in the usual intake distributions meeting the intake goals. As discussed previously, designing menu offerings to meet intake targets is a dif-

TABLE 5-2 Identification of the Target Median Intake[a] of Vitamin B_6 to Obtain a 10 Percent Prevalence of Inadequacy in Older Women

Study[b]	EAR (mg/day)	Intake at 10th Percentile (mg/day)	Difference (EAR − intake at 10th percentile)	Median Intake (mg/day)	Target Median Intake (mg/day)
CSFII	1.3	0.88	0.42	1.41	1.83
NHANES III	1.3	1.04	0.26	1.53	1.79
Boston	1.3	0.6	0.7	1.0	1.70

[a] The target median intake is estimated by adding the difference between the Estimated Average Requirement (EAR) and the intake at the acceptable prevalence of inadequacy (in this case, 10%) to the observed median intake.
[b] CSFII = Continuing Survey of Food Intakes by Individuals, NHANES III = Third National Health and Nutrition Examination Survey, Boston = Boston Diet Study. SOURCE: IOM (1998a).

ficult task. Meals with an average nutrient content equal to the median of the target usual nutrient intake distribution may not meet the planning goals, as individuals in a group tend to consume less than what is offered and served to them. Thus, the planner might aim for a menu that offers a choice of meals with a nutrient content range that includes, or even exceeds, the median of the target usual nutrient intake distribution.

Step 4. Assess implementation of the plan.

Ideally, after the menu has been planned and implemented, a survey would be conducted to assess intakes and determine whether the planning goal has been attained. This would then be used as the basis for further planning.

PLANNING MENUS FOR A SCHOOL NUTRITION PROGRAM

Probably the largest group planning application in the United States is for the nutrition assistance programs sponsored by the U.S. Department of Agriculture (USDA). These include the Food Stamp Program; the Supplemental Nutrition Program for Women, Infants, and Children; the Child and Adult Care Feeding Program; the National School Lunch Program (NSLP); the School Breakfast Program (SBP); and the Summer Food Service Program.

The NSLP and SBP are federally administered nutrition programs that operate daily in the nation's schools. The primary objective of these programs is "to safeguard the health and well-being of the Nation's children" (Richard B. Russell National School Lunch Act, 42 U.S.C. § 1751(2) [2002]). The Recommended Dietary Allowances (RDAs) have long formed the basis for food-based menu planning in the school nutrition programs. USDA regulations require that NSLP lunches provide, over time, one-third of the RDA for key nutrients. The goal of the SBP is to provide one-fourth of the RDA. Findings from two school nutrition dietary assessment studies indicate that, on average, school meals meet or exceed their goals of *offering* one-third of the RDA for lunch and one-fourth of the RDA for breakfast (Burghardt et al., 1995; Devaney et al., 1995; Fox et al., 2001).[2]

---

2 It is important to note that program regulations are based on the former RDAs. In addition to the implications of the framework developed for group planning in this report, the concepts underlying the new RDAs and differences between the new and old RDAs are important considerations in planning school meals.

Thus, planning for the school nutrition programs has focused on what is offered in school meals. Since it can be assumed that the intent of the USDA programs is to protect the intakes of the target population, the following approach to planning is indicated.

Multiple program objectives for school-based meals lead to important analytic issues in applying the group-planning framework. If the objective of the school nutrition programs were simply to provide meals that would replicate what school children would get in the absence of the programs, then application of the group-planning framework discussed in Chapter 3 would not be appropriate. Planners would simply examine the distributions of usual nutrient intake at breakfast and lunch and attempt to provide school meals that would result in these same usual intake distributions.

Since the school nutrition programs, however, have nutritional objectives—such as safeguarding the health of the nation's children through the provision of nutritionally adequate meals in school (as stated in the language of the federal legislation)—then the group-planning framework developed in Chapter 3 is relevant and the question is how best to apply it. Actual application of the framework is difficult since school meals supply only part of children's usual daily intake, while Dietary Reference Intakes (DRIs) are defined on the basis of usual daily intake. USDA has addressed this issue in its current regulations that specify that school lunches and breakfasts must provide, on average, one-third and one-fourth of the RDA, respectively. However, the current practice of prorating of the RDA for meals offered does not imply that it is appropriate to prorate the DRIs for dietary planning or assessment. The DRIs are a set of dietary reference values based on nutrient intakes over a period of time and are not meant to be divided into parts of a day. In addition, the proportion of usual intake accounted for by breakfast and lunch varies considerably among individuals.

Despite these difficult conceptual issues, there are some options for applying the framework for planning school meals. The first step is to examine daily usual intakes of a representative group of children covered by the school nutrition programs. Table 5-3 presents data on the usual intakes of vitamin A, vitamin C, and zinc for boys 9 to 13 years of age from the Third National Health and Nutrition Examination Survey and the Continuing Survey of Food Intakes by Individuals (IOM, 2000b, 2001). These data suggest a low prevalence of inadequacy for the intakes of vitamin C and zinc. For vitamin A, the estimated prevalence of inadequacy is 5 to 10 percent.

Suppose planners were interested in using information on the usual intakes of school children to plan the school meals consumed

TABLE 5-3 Daily Usual Intake of Vitamins A and C and Zinc, Boys 9 to 13 Years of Age

Percentile	Vitamin A (RAE)[a] (EAR = 445 µg RAE)	Vitamin C (mg)[b] (EAR = 39 mg)	Zinc (mg)[b] (EAR = 7.0 mg)
1	311	44.1	5.4
2	350	47.9	6.0
3	377	51.7	6.3
5	415	59.2	6.9
10	480	65.9	7.7
25	606	85.6	9.1
50	774	119.3	11.2
95	1,330	334.6	18.5
99	1,635	598.3	28.5
Approximate percent < EAR	5–10%	0%	5%
Target median intake	774 + 80	—	—

[a] Usual intake from food only. Taken from the Continuing Survey of Food Intakes by Individuals and converted to retinol activity equivalents (RAE) using data on vitamin A and carotenoid intakes. EAR = Estimated Average Requirement.
[b] Usual intake from food and supplements. Taken from the Third National Health and Nutrition Examination Survey and adjusted for day-to-day variation using the Iowa State University method.
SOURCE: IOM (2000b, 2001).

by program participants. As described in Chapter 3, determining the target usual intake distribution first involves selecting a group prevalence of inadequacy. In the case of these selected nutrients, planners are likely to conclude that the usual intakes of vitamin C and zinc are adequate, and would therefore plan to maintain current intakes. For vitamin A, however, if the acceptable group prevalence of inadequacy is set at 2 to 3 percent rather than the current 5 to 10 percent, planners would aim to shift the usual intake distribution by about 80 µg retinol activity equivalents (RAE) so only 2 to 3 percent are below the EAR, resulting in a target median intake of 854 µg RAE.

The next step in applying the group-planning framework is to decide how the school nutrition programs should or could be used to achieve the targeted usual intake distribution. Two possible options are (1) to derive the target daily usual intake distribution and prorate the target intakes across meals, or (2) to derive the target daily usual intake distribution, estimate the deficit in 24-hour intakes, and plan for intakes from school meals to make up these deficits.

The first of these options is consistent with the way in which the school nutrition programs currently operate, where the amount offered in the school meals is a specified proportion of the RDAs. Implementing this option in the case of vitamin A, for example, would entail prorating the target usual intake distribution, with the target median intake of 854 µg RAE, in such a way that a certain proportion is consumed at breakfast and at lunch.

The second option makes the nutritional objectives of the school nutrition programs more explicit. Implementing this option involves planning school breakfasts and lunches such that the distribution of usual daily intakes of participants is the target usual intake distribution. In this case, the school meals are expected to make up the deficit in usual daily vitamin A intake of 80 µg RAE. The deficit could be made up by planning menus that would add 80 µg RAE to the median intake at breakfast or lunch. This amount could also be split between the two meals. Tailoring food choices or portion sizes at the point of service may be impractical. Thus, a methodology of planning for heterogeneous groups may be needed.

In summary, application of the group-planning framework for the U.S. food and nutrition assistance programs is a complex task that involves several considerations related to program goals, nutritional considerations, and program implementation. Like any new paradigm, it must first be tested for its feasibility and practicality. The discussion of the school nutrition programs above is intended to identify the main issues involved in applying the framework and options to consider in its implementation—it is not intended to prescribe how this framework should be implemented in the context of school feeding.

PLANNING DIETS FOR A HETEROGENEOUS GROUP USING A NUTRIENT DENSITY APPROACH

The examples provided to this point have assumed that planning is occurring for a group that consists of a single life stage and gender group or life stage and gender groups with similar requirements. Frequently, however, planning will occur for groups that encompass multiple life stage and gender groups with very different nutrient and energy requirements. Two examples that incorporate the nutrient density approaches described in Chapter 4 are provided below. The first illustrates the simple nutrient density approach, in which the target median intake for each subgroup is compared to the average energy needs of the subgroup. The second example illustrates the nutrient density distribution approach, which includes a consideration of the variability of energy and nutrient needs within each subgroup.

To compare and contrast the two approaches, both examples consider the vitamin C intakes of a group consisting of adolescent boys aged 14 to 18 years, women aged 19 to 50 years, and men aged 19 to 50 years. As in most of the examples in this chapter, data used here are real data, in this case collected in the 1994–1996 Continuing Survey of Food Intakes by Individuals. Intake distributions of vitamin C and of energy for the three subgroups were adjusted using the Iowa State University method (IOM, 2000a; Nusser et al., 1996). The estimated usual intake distributions of energy in each of the subgroups were used as estimates for the distributions of requirements of energy. The examples were constructed using the data presented in Table 5-4.

Simple Nutrient Density Approach

Step 1. Obtain the target median vitamin C intake for adolescent boys, adult women, and adult men.

Adolescent Boys. The estimated prevalence of vitamin C inadequacy in this particular subgroup of adolescent boys is approximately 19 percent when comparing usual intakes to their Estimated Average Requirement (EAR) of 63 mg/day. Thus, a target vitamin C intake distribution would be obtained by shifting the baseline usual intake distribution by an amount sufficient to move the 3rd percentile of the distribution from its current 31 mg to approximately 63 mg (assuming that a prevalence of inadequacy of 2 to 3 percent is what is desired). By shifting the intakes of vitamin C by 32 mg/day (EAR − 3rd percentile: 63 − 31 = 32), the target vitamin C intake distribution is obtained (as was described in Chapter 3). In this target vitamin C intake distribution, the 3rd percentile is now approximately at the EAR of 63 mg/day. The target median intake is now 139 mg/day.

Adult Women. The prevalence of inadequacy among the women in this example is approximately 33 percent compared to their EAR of 60 mg. To obtain the target vitamin C intake distribution, it is necessary to shift the distribution by approximately 37 mg/day (EAR − 3rd percentile: 60 − 23 = 37), so that the proportion of

TABLE 5-4 Usual Vitamin C and Energy Intakes of a Group Containing Three Discrete Subgroups

Subgroup	EAR[a]	n	Median	Mean	SD[b]
Usual Vitamin C Intake (mg/day)					
Boys 14–18 y	63	474	107		70
Women 19–50 y	60	2,498	77		48
Men 19–50 y	75	2,726	95		67
Usual Energy Intake (kcal/day)					
Boys 14–18 y			2,801	2,881	782
Women 19–50 y			1,685	1,719	430
Men 19–50 y			2,561	2,659	809

[a] EAR = Estimated Average Requirement.
[b] SD = standard deviation.
SOURCE: USDA/ARS (1997).

target usual intakes below the EAR of 60 mg/day is about 3 percent. The target median intake is now 114 mg/day.

Adult Men. The prevalence of inadequacy among the men in this example is approximately 35 percent based on their EAR of 75 mg. To obtain the target vitamin C intake distribution, it is necessary to shift the distribution by approximately 49 mg/day (EAR – 3rd percentile: 75 – 26 = 49), so that the proportion of target usual intakes below the EAR of 75 mg/day is now about 3 percent. The target median intake is now 144 mg/day.

Step 2. Divide the target median vitamin C intake by the mean energy intake or expenditure in each subgroup to obtain the target median nutrient intake relative to energy.

In this step, the median of the target usual intake distribution of the nutrient (vitamin C), which has been developed to exceed the requirements of most members of the group, is divided by the mean energy intake. The mean energy intake, rather than the median, is used because for energy, assuming the group (or subgroup) is in energy balance, the mean energy intake is equal to the mean energy requirement, and there are negative effects to providing energy above or below the requirement.

Percentile			
3rd	5th	95th	Prevalence of Inadequacy (%)
31	38	256	19
23	28	178	33
26	31	238	35
	1,747	4,288	
	1,071	2,248	
	1,537	4,112	

Adolescent Boys. The target median vitamin C intake for adolescent boys in this example is 139 mg/day. With a mean energy intake of 2,881 kcal/day, this leads to a target median vitamin C intake of 48.2 mg/1,000 kcal.

Adult Women. The target median vitamin C intake for adult women of 114 mg/day is divided by their mean energy intake of 1,719 kcal/day, for a target median intake of 66.3 mg/1,000 kcal.

Adult Men. The target median vitamin C intake for adult men of 144 mg/day is divided by their mean energy intake of 2,659 kcal, for a target median intake of 54.2 mg/1,000 kcal.

Step 3. Compare the target median nutrient intakes relative to energy for each discrete subgroup to identify the subgroup with the reference intake (i.e., the highest nutrient requirement relative to energy intake) and set planning goals for the whole group. Ensure that intakes of the other subgroups will not be above the Tolerable Upper Intake Level (UL).

Among these three groups, women have the highest target median vitamin C intake relative to their mean energy intake. Thus, the target reference intake for planning purposes would be 66.3 mg/1,000 kcal.

Whether the target reference intake would lead to intakes above the UL cannot be accurately determined using the simple density approach. However, an indication of the likelihood of excessive intakes can be obtained by calculating the anticipated intake at the 95th percentiles of the energy intake distribution, using the reference density. For adolescent boys, the 95th percentile of energy intake is 4,288 kcal/day, which would be associated with a vitamin C intake of 284 mg/day (4,288 kcal × 66.3 mg/1,000 kcal). This intake remains considerably below the UL of 1,800 mg/day for adolescents. Similarly, for adult men the 95th percentile of energy intake is 4,112 kcal/day, which would be associated with a vitamin C intake of 273 mg/day using the reference density. This too is well below the UL of 2,000 mg/day for adult men.

Step 4. Assess whether the plan was successfully implemented.

Ideally, after the plan has been implemented, assessment of intakes would be conducted to confirm whether the acceptable prevalence of inadequacy has been attained and whether the prevalence of intakes above the UL is low.

Nutrient Density Distribution Approach

Step 1. Obtain the target usual vitamin C intake distribution.

The first step in the nutrient density distribution approach is similar to the first step in the simple nutrient density approach. However, instead of focusing on one point of the target usual intake distribution (the median), in this case the entire distribution is of interest.

Adolescent Boys. As described in the simple nutrient density approach, the target usual vitamin C intake distribution for adolescent boys would be shifted up by 32 mg/day. This would lead to a distribution with a median intake of 139 mg/day, and 5th and 95th percentiles of 70 and 288 mg/day, respectively.

Adult Women. For adult women, the usual vitamin C intake distribution would be repositioned by 37 mg/day to obtain the target intake distribution. It would have a median of 114 mg/day and 5th and 95th percentiles of 65 and 215 mg/day, respectively.

Adult Men. The usual intake distribution for adult men would be shifted up by 49 mg/day to obtain a target intake distribution with a median of 144 mg/day, and 5th and 95th percentiles of 80 and 287 mg/day, respectively.

Step 2. Define the target usual vitamin C density intake distribution for each definable subgroup.

Given a target nutrient intake distribution and a usual energy intake distribution, it is now possible to derive the *target nutrient density intake distribution* for each subgroup. This is done by using one of the two equations presented in Chapter 4 to compute the average nutrient density intake for each individual in each subgroup (or for a sample of individuals in each subgroup). The average nutrient density intake for each individual is then combined to form the target nutrient density intake distribution for each subgroup.

In this example, an average (over a number of possible energy intake values) vitamin C density intake was computed for a random sample of 400 individuals from each of the subgroups (boys, women, men). For each individual in each subgroup sample, a random sample of 400 energy intakes was drawn from the usual energy intake distribution for that subgroup. The target vitamin C density intake was constructed using equation (2) from Chapter 4:

$$\text{Average nutrient density intake} = (1/m) \, \Sigma_{j=1}^{m} \, (\text{usual nutrient intake/energy intake}_j) \times 1{,}000$$

Equation (2) was used rather than equation (1) because the calculation was performed on a random sample of each subgroup (Monte Carlo approach) rather than the entire distribution of all possible nutrient and energy intake combinations.

This procedure was accomplished as follows:

• A random sample of 400 intakes was drawn from the target usual vitamin C intake distribution for each subgroup.
• Next, for each of those 400 vitamin C intakes in each subgroup, a random sample of 400 energy intakes was drawn from the usual energy intake distribution in the corresponding subgroup. Thus, a given vitamin C intake (e.g., 46 mg) was associated with 400 different energy intakes (e.g., 46 mg/1,750 kcal, 46 mg/3,002 kcal, 46 mg/2,222 kcal, and so on). From those 400 different densities for each nutrient intake, the average nutrient density intake was calculated using the second equation (nutrient density intake = $[1/m]\Sigma_{j=1}^{m}$ [usual nutrient intake/energy intake$_j$] $\times$ 1,000) where m is equal to 400.

• This process was repeated a total of 400 times in each subgroup (for each of the 400 vitamin C intakes in each subgroup).

• Then, for each subgroup, the 400 average nutrient density intakes were used to construct the target vitamin C density intake distribution.

Adolescent Boys. In the case of boys aged 14 to 18 years, the target nutrient density intake distribution has a median of 52 mg of vitamin C/1,000 kcal, and 5th and 95th percentiles of 26 and 112 mg/1,000 kcal, respectively.

Adult Women. In this example, the target vitamin C density intake distribution for women aged 19 to 50 years has a median of 71 mg/1,000 kcal, a 5th percentile of 42 mg/1,000 kcal, and a 95th percentile of 135 mg/1,000 kcal.

Adult Men. For the subgroup of men aged 19 to 50 years, the resulting target vitamin C density intake distribution has a median of 57 mg/1,000 kcal, and 5th and 95th percentiles of 33 and 115 mg / 1,000 kcal, respectively.

Step 3. Compare the target median vitamin C density for each discrete subgroup to set planning goals for the group as a whole.

In this example, the target vitamin C density distribution for women had the highest median (71 mg/1,000 kcal compared to 57 mg/1,000 kcal for adult men and 52 mg/1,000 kcal for adolescent boys). This amount would normally be chosen as the reference nutrient density intake distribution for the group as a whole, and intakes would be planned on this basis. The planned menus resulting from this activity should be checked for both total milligrams of vitamin C and milligrams of vitamin C/1,000 kcal.

Comparison of the Simple Nutrient Density Approach and the Nutrient Density Distribution Approach

It is useful to compare the planning results that would be achieved when using the two nutrient density methods described above (and in Chapter 4). Recall that for the same group of boys, women, and men, the median of the target nutrient density intake distribution that would be obtained by simply dividing the target median vitamin C intake by the mean energy requirement in each of the groups was 48, 66, and 54 mg/1,000 kcal, respectively. Based on these values, the planner would aim for a target nutrient density intake distribution in each of the subgroups with a median equal to the highest of the three values, or 66 mg/1,000 kcal. Using this method, which does not take into account the distribution of energy requirements in the group, results in a prevalence of vitamin C inadequacy of approximately 8 to 9 percent for the women in the group (for adolescent boys and men the resulting intakes would be adequate for all individuals). In contrast, using the nutrient density distribution approach results in a projected prevalence of inadequacy of approximately 2 to 3 percent for the women, and essentially zero for the men and adolescent boys. Because the nutrient density distribution approach accounts for variability in energy intakes, it is more likely to achieve planning goals.

INTERVENTIONS THAT MAY CHANGE THE SHAPE OF THE INTAKE DISTRIBUTION: NUTRIENT SUPPLEMENTATION

Some planning applications involve interventions that aim to modify food or nutrient intakes. One way to modify nutrient intakes when a food-based approach is not possible is to incorporate use of a nutrient supplement within a group. If every individual in the group consumed the identical supplement every day, the distribution of usual intakes would simply shift up, with no change in shape, by the dose of the supplement. In practice, however, all individuals in a group may not take the supplement on a regular basis, and, among those who do take it, the dose may not be constant. As a result, misleading conclusions and practices may result if uniform supplement usage is assumed.

As an example, suppose a planner wished to reduce the predicted prevalence of zinc inadequacy among a group of free-living teenage girls through the use of a supplement. The first step would be to examine the current intake distribution. Let us assume that the group of teenage girls being targeted is similar to the sample of girls aged 14 to 18 years surveyed by the Third National Health and Nutrition Examination Survey (NHANES III), so that data from NHANES III can be used to estimate the current intake distribution. Participants in NHANES III are free-living and have not been the target of any national public health intervention regarding the use of zinc supplements. Table 5-5 presents information on the distribution of usual intake of zinc from foods (adjusted for within-person variation) and from supplements. The EAR for zinc in girls aged 14 to 18 years has been set at 7.3 mg/day. As shown in Table 5-5, more than 25 percent of teen girls had inadequate usual intake of zinc from food alone. If the acceptable group risk of inad-

TABLE 5-5 Estimated Usual Zinc Intake Distribution for Girls, 14 to 18 Years of Age (mg/day)

Percentile of Usual Intake	Zinc from Foods	Zinc from Supplements	Total Zinc[a]
1	4.0	0.83	3.9
3	4.7	0.9	4.8
5	5.1	1.0	5.2
10	5.8	1.0	5.8
25	7.1	2.5	7.2
50	8.8	8.0	9.0
75	10.9	15.0	11.6
90	13.2	15.0	13.8
95	16.4	37.5	16.0
99	18.6	45.5	26.6
Sample size	949	48	949
Mean	9.27	9.75	9.82

[a] Because only 48 of the 949 girls used supplements containing zinc, total zinc intake does not equal the sum of the zinc intakes from food and supplements.
SOURCE: IOM (2001).

equacy were set at 3 percent, then the 3rd percentile of usual intake should be increased to the level of the Estimated Average Requirement (EAR). That is, the 3rd percentile value of 4.7 in Table 5-5 should increase to 7.3, an increase of 2.6 mg. Assuming that the usual intake distribution does not change its shape, the median intake would be the existing median intake + 2.6 mg (8.8 mg + 2.6 mg = 11.4 mg). This new usual intake distribution could be achieved if everyone took a supplement containing 2.6 mg of zinc.

Before recommending consumption of a supplement containing 2.6 mg of zinc, however, it is important to determine current supplement use. Accordingly, the next step is to examine the reported use of zinc supplements and the computed distribution of intakes from both sources, which are shown in Table 5-5. Note that only 48 of the 949 teen girls in the survey reported taking a zinc supplement (approximately 5 percent), so including supplements does not affect the total intake for most participants. Indeed, the distribution of total zinc intake differs primarily in the upper percentiles, with very little change in the lower percentiles. The third percentile increases only 0.1 mg/day, from 4.7 to 4.8 mg/day. Thus, there is almost no effect of current use of zinc supplements on the predicted prevalence of inadequacy. The increase that is needed to reduce the prevalence to 3 percent is now 2.5 mg/day (7.3 – 4.8) versus 2.6 mg/day when food alone is considered.

In theory, planners could develop an education intervention that recommended that teen girls consume a supplement that provides 2.5 mg of zinc/day. Special supplements providing this level of intake could even be marketed. However, several observations regarding supplement usage patterns in free-living populations are important to highlight:

• Although the average supplement provided 9.75 mg of zinc, the change in the median intake of zinc, when adding in supplement use, was only 0.2 mg (9.0 mg – 8.8 mg).
• Although the median intake of zinc increased by 0.2 mg when supplements were included, the magnitude of the change at the 3rd percentile was only 0.1 mg.
• The prevalence of inadequate intake of zinc still exceeds 25 percent, even when intake from currently consumed supplements is added to the intake from food.
• As is usually the case, supplement usage was not uniform across this group of individuals. Teen girls with higher intakes of zinc from food were more likely to take a supplement and perhaps more likely to take a higher-dose supplement.

Thus, supplement use by a free-living population may not achieve the planner's goals, and the challenge is to determine how to either shift the whole distribution by 2.5 mg/day or to increase the use of supplements or zinc-rich foods by individuals in the lower percentiles. If an additional supplement of 2.5 mg/day of zinc was distributed *and consumed* by the entire population, then the distribution would shift as desired. As the data in Table 5-5 illustrate, it may take an intensive intervention to achieve this goal.

An alternative approach is to ensure supplement use by those in the lower percentiles. This might be possible if there are characteristics that would identify individuals with low intakes (such as income level or age). Such interventions to increase supplement use are likely to be more successful in a confined population (where supplement use could be monitored) than in a free-living one.

The important conclusion from this example of planning is that an intervention to change usual intakes through supplementation can be difficult to design and implement. In a free-living population, not every person can be expected to consistently take a supplement (or a given food or food group rich in a specific nutrient), and interventions in such a group may be expected to change both the location and shape of the usual intake distribution. It is important to understand the patterns and predictors of supplement use in order to model and plan such interventions. Simply assuming uniform use of a supplement in free-living populations would likely result in a failure to achieve the planning goals.

FOOD FORTIFICATION

Fortification is often seen as a potentially desirable public health measure that could achieve an increased intake of specified nutrients without changes in food consumption practices or compliance with specific nutrient supplement usage. Historically, mandatory fortification programs have been applied in many countries as a means to address particular public health concerns. In these programs, public health authorities determine both the food vehicles and levels of fortification, and only fortified versions of the selected foods are permitted on the market. One such example is the mandatory fortification of table salt with iodine in Canada, a measure undertaken to reduce iodine deficiency in the population. Alternatively, food fortification programs may be voluntary, with food manufacturers having the option of adding particular nutrients (sometimes within prescribed limits) to foods, but not being required to do so. One example of this approach is the fortification of orange juice with calcium; because the program is voluntary, it is possible to purchase orange juice with or without calcium added. Regulations on food fortification differ between Canada and the United States, with voluntary fortification permitted in the United States.

Regardless of whether fortification is mandatory or voluntary, if it is intended to achieve public health goals, then it is often necessary to "target" the fortification. Such targeting could be accomplished by selecting only foods for fortification that are used exclusively or in substantially greater amounts by the group targeted by a fortification program, or by mounting an educational program to promote the use of specific fortified foods by the target group.

Fortification, however, also carries the potential for detrimental effects. Fortification of foods might increase nutrient intakes to excessive levels among those persons who have high intakes of the fortified food or those who already have high intakes of the nutrient and then consume the newly fortified food. Minimally controlled fortification of foods, even at low levels in individual foods, can have unexpected effects, ranging from negligible benefits to public health concerns about potentially detrimental high intakes. Further, unless fortified foods reach only the target group (unusual in practice, except for infant foods), it is possible that the risk of detrimental effects will appear in other sectors of the population (i.e., nontarget groups). Because of the range of potential effects that can accompany fortification programs, both beneficial and detrimental, the potential impact of proposed fortification is usually examined before implementation.

In general, no simple method can be used to predict the effects of fortification. Fortifying foods with nutrients will have impacts on the nutrient intakes of those who consume the fortified foods and will not have impacts on those who do not consume them. Further, the degree of impact depends not only on the level of the nutrient added, but also on the distribution of usual intakes of the food. In recent years, predicting the effect of fortification has been complicated in the United States by introduction of food products fortified with a nutrient while the evaluation of the need for fortification is still in progress. Thus, it is difficult to anticipate changes in the usual intake distribution of the nutrient when even changes in the *amount* of the nutrient in the food supply are almost impossible to predict. A more extended discussion on the issue of voluntary fortification is presented in Appendix D.

The approach presented below involves modeling and estimating the effects of a mock fortification effort by using data on foods and nutrients consumed and then calculating the change in nutrient intake after the foods are fortified. The predicted benefits and risks associated with the fortification can be assessed through application of assessment methods based on the Estimated Average Requirement (EAR) and Tolerable Upper Intake Level (UL) (IOM, 2000a).

Such an approach was utilized by Lewis and colleagues (1999) to examine the impact of folate fortification of cereal-grain products in the United States if increased fortification of foods was mandated. A similar approach is illustrated below for the hypothetical addition of vitamin A to fluid milk. For simplicity, this example assumes that only one food will be fortified with vitamin A. As was discussed earlier, this assumption is unlikely to hold when voluntary fortification of foods with vitamin A is permitted.

Addition of Vitamin A to Fluid Milk

Two levels of requirements for vitamin A have been established with different functional endpoints in mind (IOM, 2001). For adult women, the EAR for prevention of functional deficiency of vitamin A is 300 μg retinol activity equivalents (RAE)/day while the EAR to establish and maintain desirable levels of liver vitamin A stores has been set at 500 µg RAE/day. For adult women 19 to 50 years of age, examination of the 1994–1996 CSFII (USDA/ARS, 1997) data suggests that about 15 percent have intakes below 300 µg RAE/day and hence have intakes apparently inadequate to meet their own functional requirements. The same data suggest that about 44 percent may have intakes inadequate to provide minimal stores of vitamin A. These descriptors of a potential problem may motivate planning interventions to raise vitamin A intakes in this target group, although planners would also obtain other types of data (e.g., biochemical or clinical outcome information such as incidence of night blindness) before proceeding with an intervention.

Suppose that in order to increase vitamin A intake by adult women, a fortification program is considered that adds vitamin A to all fluid milk. In the United States milk is frequently fortified with vitamin A, but it is not required. This example assumes that no fortification is currently taking place.

Based on data from the CSFII (USDA/ARS, 1997), Table 5-6 illustrates the predicted impact of this fortification on the distribution of total vitamin A intake of adult women. Total intake equals reported

TABLE 5-6 Impact of the Addition of Vitamin A to Milk on the Expected Distribution of Total Vitamin A Intake in Women 19–50 Years of Age

Percentile of Intake	Level of Addition of Vitamin A (as Retinyl Ester) to Fluid Milk (µg/100 ml)						
	0	50	100	150	200	250	300
1	135	138	140	143	145	147	149
5	225	238	247	253	259	268	276
10	272	287	298	308	319	327	337
25	368	398	421	445	465	484	505
50	542	592	635	670	711	747	787
75	785	872	964	1,083	1,151	1,245	1,333
90	1,150	1,259	1,389	1,549	1,679	1,811	1,954
95	1,390	1,560	1,715	1,915	2,084	2,234	2,411
99	2,026	2,154	2,372	2,573	2,777	3,067	3,325

NOTE: n = 2,325 women. In this example, the amount by which vitamin A increases reflects the initial fluid milk consumption of those in the various percentile groups. For example, those in the 1st percentile drink little milk, so their vitamin A intake increases only slightly as the level of addition of vitamin A to milk increases. In contrast, those in the 99th percentile, who drink much more milk, have a much greater increase.
SOURCE: USDA/ARS (1997) as reported in IOM (2001).

intake of vitamin A plus the increase that would come from consuming fortified milk. It is possible to determine the theoretical increase because the CSFII database can be disaggregated to determine the amount of milk consumed by each individual. Thus, the amount of the increase in vitamin A intake will reflect the amount of milk consumed: those women who consume large amounts of fluid milk will increase their intake substantially, while those who consume little or no fluid milk will not increase their intake.

Table 5-7 provides some information on the likely benefits and potential risks of this fortification. Based on the results for adult women, adding vitamin A to fluid milk could be expected to have beneficial impacts by raising intakes without a major concern about possible detrimental effects. That is, as the level of fortification increases, the prevalence of usual intake of vitamin A less than the EAR to prevent night blindness (300 µg RAE) declines from approximately 15 percent at no fortification to approximately 7 percent at a fortification level of 300 µg of retinol/100 mL of milk. The prevalence of usual intake less than the EAR for maintaining stores (500 µg RAE) declines from 44 percent at no fortification to 24

TABLE 5-7 Apparent Benefits and Potential Risks Associated with the Addition of Vitamin A to all Fluid Milk as a Function of Level of Addition, Women 19–50 Years of Age

Level of Addition[a] (µg/100 ml)	Prevalence of Inadequate Intakes[b] (below the EAR)		Prevalence of Potentially Excessive Intakes[c]
	% < EAR (300 µg RAE)	% < EAR (500 µg RAE)	% > UL (3,000 µg)
0 (baseline)	14.6	44.3	0.0
50	12.1	38.9	0.0
100	10.2	35.6	0.1
150	8.8	33.3	0.1
200	8.0	29.9	0.2
250	7.6	28.8	0.3
300	6.9	24.3	0.7

NOTE: n = 2,325 women.
[a] Added as a retinyl ester.
[b] Based on total vitamin A intake as µg of retinol activity equivalents (RAE). EAR = Estimated Average Requirement.
[c] Based on preformed vitamin A only. UL = Tolerable Upper Intake Level.
SOURCE: USDA/ARS (1997).

percent at a fortification level of 300 µg of retinol/100 ml of milk. In contrast, as the level of fortification increases, the prevalence of usual intake above the UL increases only slightly from 0 to 0.7 percent. On the basis of this evidence only, the decision to fortify milk with vitamin A would seem a worthwhile endeavor.

Other subgroups, however, may not have the same benefits or risks at that level of vitamin A fortification. Table 5-8 shows the impact of this fortification of fluid milk for boys 9 to 13 years of age. In this case, the prevalence of inadequate vitamin A intake without fortification (at baseline) is lower than for adult women. With fortification, the prevalence of inadequate intakes based on maintaining stores (EAR = 445 µg RAE for this age group) declines from about 11 percent to 3.5 percent. Since there is very little prevalence of inadequate intake of vitamin A based on preventing night blindness (EAR = 230 µg RAE for this age group) without fortification, the addition of more vitamin A to milk would have a negligible effect on prevalence of this criterion of inadequate intake. On the other hand, the potential detrimental effect with fortification is

TABLE 5-8 Apparent Benefits and Potential Risks Associated with the Addition of Vitamin A to all Fluid Milk as a Function of Level of Addition, Boys 9–13 Years of Age

Level of Addition[a] µg/100 ml	Prevalence of Inadequate Intakes[b] (below the EAR)		Prevalence of Potentially Excessive Intakes[c]
	% < EAR (230 µg RAE)	% < EAR (445 µg RAE)	% > UL (1,700 µg)
0 (baseline)	0.5	11.1	0.9
50	0.3	8.2	2.6
100	0.3	7.0	5.9
150	0.3	5.6	12.2
200	0.3	4.5	19.0
250	0.3	4.2	30.0
300	0.3	3.5	37.8

NOTE: n = 574 boys.
[a] Added as a retinyl ester.
[b] Based on total vitamin A intake as µg of retinol activity equivalents (RAE). EAR = Estimated Average Requirement.
[c] Based on preformed vitamin A only. UL = Tolerable Upper Intake Level.
SOURCE: USDA/ARS (1997).

high, as shown by increasing percentages with usual intake above the UL as the level of fortification increases. Specifically, with no fortification, the prevalence of usual intakes above the UL for this age group is approximately 1 percent, while at a fortification level of 300 µg of retinol/100 mL of milk, the prevalence of usual intakes above the UL would increase to 38 percent. The reason for these differential impacts for adult women and boys 9 to 13 years of age is that the latter group has a higher initial intake of vitamin A, and an overall higher consumption of the vehicle chosen for fortification—milk.

By combining the analyses for adult women and boys 9 to 13 years of age, the relationship between the potential benefits to women and the potential risks to adolescent boys of fortifying milk at the various levels is demonstrated. Figure 5-1 summarizes the benefits to adult women by the declining percentage with inadequate intake and the increasing potential risk to boys 9 to 13 years of age by the increasing percentage over the UL. Based on these results, planners would have to consider the predicted potential risk to boys 9 to 13 years of age and the predicted benefits to the target group of adult women before reaching a decision on whether to fortify and at what

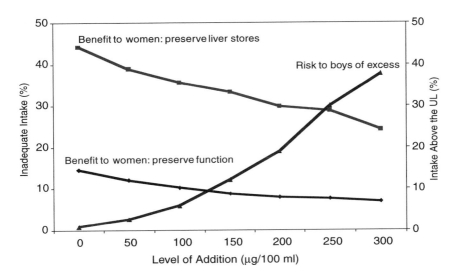

FIGURE 5-1 Projected benefits and potential risk associated with the addition of vitamin A to fluid milk. UL = Tolerable Upper Intake Level.

amount. Of course, this exercise should be repeated for other subgroups of the population before final decisions are made.

When only a few foods are involved in compulsory fortification, regulatory agencies run mock fortification studies (like the vitamin A example above) and weigh the expected benefits and potential risks associated with different levels of fortification. However, with voluntary fortification such as what is currently the practice in the United States, as the number of fortified foods increases, it becomes extremely difficult to run meaningful mock fortification scenarios. In addition, it has not been possible to keep food composition databases current with regard to brand-specific fortified foods, and not all nutrient composition databases in the United States are designed to do so. Food composition databases in the United States used in national surveys usually reflect the average composition of foods that are available in the market, with varieties or brands weighted by general market share. Thus, it is difficult to investigate the effect of voluntary fortification of specific brands of foods unless all brands within a category are fortified. More detailed survey data, as well as more specific food composition tables, are needed for investigation of brand-specific fortification.

Planning Fortification: General Conclusion and Recommendation

The principal conclusion drawn from this fortification application is the importance of examining the potential impacts on all groups—not just on the targeted subgroups that have a higher than desired prevalence of inadequate intakes without fortification. It is recommended that a modeling approach, such as that presented here, be conducted prior to any major introduction of fortification.

6

Special Considerations and Adjustments

SUMMARY

This chapter provides a discussion of the process and criteria used to establish the Dietary Reference Intakes (DRIs) in order to help users make informed judgments during the dietary planning process.

The limitations in the data used to develop the DRIs and the relationship between dietary nutrient inadequacy and inadequate nutritional status are important considerations when planning diets. This chapter also addresses factors such as nutrient bioavailability and physiological, lifestyle, and health factors that may alter nutrient requirements and lead to adjustments in the DRI values when planning dietary intakes for individuals and groups.

INTRODUCTION

It is well established that biological variability exists among individuals with regard to both nutrient requirements and susceptibility to adverse effects from excessive nutrient intakes. These individual differences, when known, in the normal, apparently healthy population have already been considered in establishing the Dietary Reference Intakes (DRIs). Specifically, variability in individual requirements around the Estimated Average Requirement (EAR) is considered in setting the Recommended Dietary Allowance (RDA), the intake recommendation for individuals. The Adequate Intake (AI) is set at a level thought to meet or exceed the needs of almost all individuals of a given life stage and gender group. The Tolerable Upper Intake Level (UL) is set at an intake at which all but the most sensitive members of a population would not be expected to experience adverse effects. Thus, most normal sources of variability have already been considered in setting the DRI values, as they apply to the typical diets of apparently healthy people in the United States and Canada. However, there are other identifiable factors that may alter nutrient requirements systematically such that the DRI values may need to be adjusted when planning nutrient intakes for certain individuals or groups. These factors, discussed below, include characteristics of the nutrient source that influence nutrient bioavailability, as well as physiological, health, or lifestyle characteristics of individuals that may require tailoring of requirement estimates.

INFLUENCE OF THE NUTRIENT SOURCES

Bioavailability

Information on the bioavailability of nutrients from foods, fortified foods, and supplemental nutrient sources has been used in developing the Dietary Reference Intakes (DRIs) and must also be considered in applying the DRIs to dietary planning. Issues regarding bioavailability for each nutrient are discussed briefly below and in greater detail in the individual DRI nutrient reports (IOM, 1997, 1998a, 2000b, 2001, 2002a).

Different sources of a nutrient can vary in chemical or physical form, which can affect bioavailability. Thus, in planning diets for individuals or groups, consideration may need to be given to whether the nutrient is supplied in its natural food matrix, as a fortificant to a food source, or in a supplemental form not associated with food. For example, U.S. Department of Agriculture food composition data have only recently been modified to reflect the different bioavailability between natural food sources of folate (1 dietary folate equivalent [DFE] = 1 μg of folate found naturally in food) and folate added as a fortificant to foods (1 DFE = 0.6 μg). Accordingly, in planning to increase an individual's folate intake by about 100 DFEs to meet the Recommended Dietary Allowance (RDA), it would be necessary to consider whether to increase the intake of fruits and vegetables or fortified grain products (or both). An increase of 100 DFEs would require 100 μg of folate from fruits and vegetables, but only 60 μg from fortified grain products. However, if the food composition data were reported in DFE units, differences in bioavailability would already have been taken into account.

The source of a nutrient can also affect the potential risk of nutrient intakes that exceed the Tolerable Upper Intake Level (UL). For several nutrients, there is no known risk of excessive intake from natural foods. Accordingly, the UL for nutrients such as magnesium, folate, niacin, and vitamin E are based only on chemical or synthetic forms obtained from supplements or added to foods (IOM 1997, 1998a, 2000b). Excessive intakes for other nutrients such as calcium, selenium, iron, and vitamins C and D are based on the combination of intakes from food and supplements (IOM 1997, 2000b, 2001).

For some nutrients, the chemical form varies within natural foods, as well as between natural and synthetic sources. For instance, heme iron, the form of approximately 40 percent of the iron in meat, poultry, and fish (Monsen et al., 1978), is generally better absorbed than the remaining (nonheme) form of iron in foods. This difference between heme and nonheme iron absorption, which is one factor that can contribute to the lower iron absorption seen in plant-based diets, has been addressed by recommending intakes for vegetarians that reflect the lower average absorption.

These differences between sources of a nutrient can be of such importance that, in some cases, it is specified which source should be used to meet nutrient intake recommendations. For example, because about 10 to 30 percent of older adults have reduced gastric acidity, they may not readily absorb the protein-bound form of vitamin B_{12} that is found naturally in food sources. To ensure that adequate vitamin B_{12} is absorbed when planning for individuals or groups where the average age is over 50, planners are encouraged to include foods fortified with vitamin B_{12} or a supplement containing vitamin B_{12} since the synthetic form of the vitamin is absorbed effectively even in those with low gastric acid secretion. Another example relates to planning for individuals or groups where women are in their childbearing years. In this case, the diet plan should include 400 µg of folate from fortified foods or supplements in addition to the food folate contained in a varied diet since studies that showed reduced risk of neural tube defects were conducted with 400 µg of folate as supplements.

Interactions with Other Nutrients, Food Components, and Properties of the Dietary Matrix

In addition to the bioavailability factors discussed above, nutrient utilization can be influenced by interactions with other nutrients or food constituents. Examples include enhancement of nonheme iron absorption by ascorbic acid; inhibition of calcium, iron, and zinc absorption by phytic acid from whole grains, nuts, and legumes; enhancement of the absorption of the fat-soluble vitamins A, D, E, and K by dietary fat; improved absorption of β-carotene in some vegetables after cooking and blending; and competitive imbalances of minerals such as calcium, iron, zinc, and copper (Mertz et al., 1994). Excessive intake of one nutrient may interfere with absorption, excretion, transport, storage, function, or metabolism of another.

Specific nutrient interactions with food components and drugs have also been identified (IOM, 1997, 1998a, 2000b, 2001, 2002a). Because of quantitative and bioavailability differences, nutrient–nutrient interactions are of particular concern in diet planning when nutrients are provided by supplementation or fortification rather than by food sources. Such interactions have been considered in setting the DRIs, including the establishment of ULs that may be specific for nutrients used in fortification or taken as supplements. Accordingly, in most cases planners do not need to make adjustments to DRIs based on nutrient–nutrient interactions.

Special Considerations for Vegetarian Diets

Well-planned vegetarian diets are associated with good health (Messina and Burke, 1997). However, not all vegetarian diets are the same. Depending on the foods included or excluded from the diet, careful planning may be required to meet recommendations for various nutrients.

For example, vitamin B_{12} is found only in foods derived from animal sources or in those foods to which it is added during fortification. Individuals following vegan diets (exclusively composed of plant foods) will need to either use a vitamin B_{12} supplement or consume fortified foods containing sufficient amounts of synthetic vitamin B_{12}. Vegetarians who do not use fluid milk are likely to have low vitamin D intakes, especially those living in northern latitudes where exposure to ultraviolet light does not occur during winter months (Ladizesky et al., 1995; Webb et al., 1988). Populations who do not use milk and milk products are likely to need additional sources of calcium in their diets. This can be achieved with the judicious selection of plant sources or the use of calcium-fortified foods and beverages.

Individuals or groups who follow vegetarian diet plans that omit all animal products are likely to be at risk for inadequate intakes of iron and zinc, which also needs to be taken into account when planning diets. Hunt and Roughead (1999) demonstrated that iron absorption from vegetarian diets was reduced compared with an omnivorous diet. In similar studies, zinc absorption was approximately 35 percent less from a lactoovovegetarian diet as compared with an omnivorous diet (Hunt et al., 1998). The description of the recommended intakes for iron and zinc further reviews the evidence of lower bioavailability of these nutrients from plant sources and recommends iron intakes for vegetarians that are higher than the RDAs for the general population (IOM, 2001).

Another nutrient of potential concern for vegetarians is protein. Because protein intakes of vegetarians are typically lower than intakes of those following omnivorous diets, the issue of protein quality becomes particularly important. In the past there were no recommended intakes for indispensable amino acids, and it was assumed that individuals consuming a mixed diet (animal and vegetable proteins with a biological value of 75 percent) with the recommended amounts of protein would obtain the needed amounts of indispensable amino acids. Now that both Estimated Average Requirements (EARs) and RDAs have been provided for indispensable amino acids, it is important to reexamine this issue.

It appears that diets adequate in total protein may not be necessarily adequate in all the indispensable amino acids, at least for lysine. Data in Table 6-1 compare the amino acid composition of various protein sources to the Food and Nutrition Board/Institute of Medicine amino acid scoring pattern (IOM, 2002a). The scoring pattern indicates the amounts of each indispensable amino acid per gram of protein needed to meet the EAR for the indispensable amino acid when total protein intake equals the EAR. A single scoring pattern has been adopted because there are relatively small differences between the amino acid requirements of children and adults when the requirements are expressed relative to total protein requirements. The data suggest that although most protein sources provide recommended amounts of threonine, tryptophan, and sulfur-containing amino acids, this may not be true for lysine. Animal protein sources provide relatively high amounts of lysine, so individuals who do not consume animal protein sources (or who consume limited amounts) may be unlikely to obtain the recommended amounts of lysine when total protein intake is limited to the RDA, unless beans are the primary protein source in their diet. Even then, diets may be marginal, as the data in the table are not adjusted for the lower digestibility often seen in plant protein sources. Therefore, in addition to planning total protein intakes, it may be necessary to plan for intakes of lysine in vegan diets.

TABLE 6-1 Selected Indispensable Amino Acid Content of
Protein Sources[a] Compared to Recommended Levels

	Indispensable Amino Acid (mg/g protein)			
	Lysine	Threonine	Tryptophan	Methionine + Cysteine
FNB/IOM scoring pattern[b]	51	27	7	25
Beef, lean	83	44	11	37
Cheddar cheese	76	33	12	29
Egg	70	49	16	56
Tofu	66	41	16	27
Soymilk	65	41	16	32
Garbanzo beans	67	37	10	26
Almonds	29[c]	32	15	25
Peanut butter	36[c]	34	10	33
Brown rice	38[c]	37	13	35
Cornmeal	28[c]	38	7	39
Wheat bread	28[c]	30	13	39

[a] USDA Nutrient Database for Standard Reference, Release 15, August 2002.
[b] From IOM (2002). The scoring patterns indicate the amounts of essential amino acids per gram of protein needed to meet the Estimated Average Requirement (EAR) for the essential amino acid when total protein intake equals the EAR for protein.
[c] The protein source would not provide recommended amounts of the indispensable amino acid if it were the only source of protein in the diet.

The need to plan intakes of lysine is likely of greatest importance for individuals whose diets emphasize plant foods *and* are relatively low in total protein. For example, the RDA for total protein for the reference 57-kg woman is 46 g/day. If she followed a plant-based diet and ate no more than the RDA of 46 g of protein daily, she would be unlikely to meet her RDA for lysine (2.2 g/day) unless 50 percent or more of her dietary protein was provided from beans or tofu (rich sources of lysine). To be specific, 23 g of protein from beans and tofu would provide about 1.5 g of lysine, and 23 g of protein from other sources, such as wheat, rice, and nuts, would provide about 0.7 g of lysine. However, if her total protein intake was greater (e.g., about 63 g/day, or similar to the median protein intake reported by women in the 1994–1996 Continuing Survey of Food Intakes by Individuals [USDA/ARS, 1997]), she could meet her RDA for lysine with much smaller amounts of beans and tofu (providing about 10 percent of her total dietary protein). Thus, planning for individuals who consume only plant sources of protein should involve careful review of lysine intakes. If their total protein intake is limited to the RDA for protein, beans and legumes should be emphasized as the major source of dietary protein.

INDIVIDUAL CHARACTERISTICS THAT INFLUENCE DIETARY REQUIREMENTS

Recommended Dietary Allowances (RDAs) and Adequate Intakes (AIs) are used as goals for nutrient intakes to meet the known nutrient requirements of almost all healthy individuals in various life stage and gender groups. As discussed below, the Dietary Reference Intake (DRI) process has already accounted for normal individual variability, and individual adjustments for factors such as age, nutrient status, genetic variation, or body size are generally not required. In other instances, adjustments may be warranted for individuals with lifestyle differences or who are ill.

Nutrient Status

Nutrient absorption, excretion, and utilization can all be substantially affected by the nutrient status of the individual (e.g., low, moderate, or high tissue concentrations). Individuals with lower body stores or who have adapted to lower intakes of a nutrient are likely to have greater rates of absorption and lower rates of excretion. These relationships have probably been best characterized in humans for iron. However, the Estimated Average Requirement (EAR) and resulting RDA are based on 18 percent iron absorption by people with minimal iron stores (defined as a serum ferritin level of 15 µg/L) and have already been adjusted for individual variation in iron status; thus, no further adjustments are required.

Genetic Variation

Rapidly expanding information on the human genome indicates many possible interactions between individual genetic traits and nutrient requirements. Examples of genetic disorders requiring nutritional treatment include classical inborn errors of metabolism such as phenylketonuria, lipoprotein lipase deficiency, and vitamin D-dependent rickets. More subtle genetic differences may contribute to variability in requirements within populations generally regarded as normal and healthy. For example, a genetic polymorphism under current investigation adversely affects homocysteine concentrations (and thus potential heart disease risk) in subjects with relatively poor folate status (Jacques et al., 1996). The continuing discovery and evaluation of genetic influences on nutritional requirements may lead to more specific recommendations for subgroups of the population. In the meantime, however, the RDAs are expected to meet the needs of almost all individuals, which should include many who may have higher than average requirements.

Unusual Body Size or Composition, Energy Expenditure, or Physical Activity

By establishing EARs and using the estimated variability of the requirement distribution to set RDAs to include 97 to 98 percent of all individuals in a life stage and gender group, these recommended intakes already account for typical variation in body size or energy expenditure in a specific group. Depending on the function and tissue distribution of the nutrient, such variation may be associated with skeletal mass, lean body mass, body water, or total body mass (IOM, 1997, 2000b). Larger individuals would be expected to have greater requirements based on larger body nutrient pools or functional compartments. Although reference body sizes (IOM, 1997) have been considered in deriving recommended intakes for specific life stage and gender subgroups, information on most nutrients is inadequate to precisely set recommendations in relation to an individual's body size or energy expenditure.

While there was insufficient evidence to define a relationship between energy requirements or body size and the requirements for thiamin, riboflavin, and niacin (IOM, 1998a), the functions of these nutrients are known to be directly related to energy metabolism. If, when planning diets, professionals choose to make an upward adjustment of B vitamin recommendations for individuals with unusually high energy requirements, the conservative approach (in terms of making recommendations to minimize the possibility of dietary inadequacy) would be to assume that vitamin requirements increase in direct proportion to energy requirements. An example of how these adjustments should be made has been provided in the DRI assessment report (IOM, 2000a).

Research on the impact of physical activity on nutrient requirements was evaluated as part of the DRI process, especially in relation to the requirements for B vitamins, vitamins with antioxidant properties such as vitamins C and E, and protein. For most nutrients, the data were considered insufficient to recommend specific alterations in the EARs or RDAs related to physical activity or athletic performance. An exception is iron. Body iron losses appear to increase with vigorous exercise, perhaps because of increased gastrointestinal blood losses or because of erythrocyte rupture within the foot during running (IOM, 2001). Consequently, athletes engaged in regular intense exercise may have average requirements for iron that range from 30 to 70 percent above those of normally active individuals. Additionally, athletes with extremely high energy intakes (exceeding 6,000 kcal/day) may have dietary phosphorus intakes that exceed the Tolerable Upper Intake Level (UL), but this is not thought to be harmful (IOM, 1997).

Age and Physiological Stage

Children

Recommended intakes change considerably across some age boundaries in children. For example, the RDA for magnesium for children ages 4 to 8 years is 130 mg/day, whereas the RDA for children ages 9 to 13 years is 240 mg/day. Clearly, magnesium needs do not change abruptly on a child's ninth birthday. Although it might appear reasonable to speculate that those at the higher end of an age range would have higher requirements than those at the lower end of the age range, in most cases knowledge of exactly how a child's nutrient requirements change with age is imprecise. For this reason, adjustment of recommended intakes within an age range is not recommended.

Adjustments in recommended intakes may be appropriate when relevant physiological changes can be identified for individuals. An example is the onset of menarche in girls. The RDA for iron for girls 14 to 18 years of age allows for iron losses in menses. If menarche occurs prior to age 14, an additional amount, about 2.5 mg of iron/day, would be needed to cover menstrual blood losses. Conversely, girls ages 14 and above who have not reached menarche can subtract 2.5 mg from the RDA for this age group. When boys or girls can be identified as undergoing the growth spurt of adolescence, the RDA for iron can be further adjusted by increasing daily intakes by 2.9 and 1.1 mg, respectively (IOM, 2001).

Women of Reproductive Age

To reduce the risk of neural tube defects it is recommended that all women capable of becoming pregnant obtain 400 µg of folate from fortified foods or supplements on a daily basis in addition to folate from a varied diet. For most women, a straightforward way to do this is to use a multivitamin supplement containing 400 µg of folate. Folate is also added to grains and cereals, but unless a highly fortified breakfast cereal is consumed, it would take unusually large amounts of some of these foods to obtain 400 µg. For example, a slice of bread contains 20 µg of added folate (the required level of folate fortification of bread).

Major differences in menstrual iron losses are an example of identifiable individual characteristics that modify nutrient requirements. These losses can be substantially modified by physiological changes such as menopause or hormonal therapy. The RDA for women ages 31 to 50 is intended to cover losses associated with menstruation, while the RDA for women over age 50 assumes that menopause has occurred. Menopause, then, rather than turning 50, is the physiologically significant event related to iron requirements. A woman who experiences menopause before age 50 (and who does not commence cyclic hormone treatment that results in the partial return of menstrual blood losses) could safely aim for an iron intake of 8 mg, the RDA for women over age 50. Conversely, a 51-year-old woman who is still menstruating regularly should aim for an iron intake of 18 mg, the RDA for women ages 31 to 50.

Dietary iron needs are lower for women using oral contraceptives due to reduced menstrual blood loss. Accordingly, the recommended intake for iron is adjusted down to 11.4 mg/day for adolescent girls and down to 10.9 mg/day for premenopausal women using oral contraceptives (IOM, 2001). Although a number of reports suggest some changes in riboflavin, B_6, or folate status for women using oral contraceptives, the available evidence does not indicate any need for adjustment in the RDAs for these nutrients.

Gestation of Multiple Fetuses

The RDAs and AIs for pregnancy and lactation have been developed for singleton pregnancies and the production of sufficient breast milk to nourish one infant. During pregnancy and lactation of multiple births, the intakes recommended for singletons may not be appropriate.

To experience good pregnancy outcomes, women who are pregnant with two or more fetuses need to gain more weight than has been associated with good outcomes for singleton pregnancies, and guidelines for weight gain during multiple pregnancies have been developed (IOM, 1990). At this point, however, average nutrient requirements for women pregnant with multiple fetuses are not known and specific recommended intakes have therefore not been derived. It has been noted, though, that intakes of some nutrients, such as protein, should be higher for women pregnant with two or more fetuses than for women pregnant with one (IOM, 2002a).

For lactating women, recommended intakes for many nutrients are developed, at least in part, on the basis of the amount of the nutrient secreted in breast milk. Women nursing two or more infants secrete greater volumes of breast milk (Saint et al., 1986); thus, it is reasonable to assume that their nutrient needs are also higher. The increased amount of energy required to nurse multiple infants will likely be met by natural appetite adjustments, and energy balance can be evaluated by monitoring body weight for mother and infants. If this increase in maternal energy intake emphasizes nutrient-dense food selections, then consumption of a variety of nutrients will be proportionally increased. Similar to pregnancy, however, specific recommendations for women nursing more than one infant have not been established.

Adults Over Age 50

For some nutrients, requirements (and thus recommendations) change in association with physiological changes that are expected to occur with aging. For example, the AI for vitamin D is higher for adults over age 50 years than for those under age 50 years.

The AI for vitamin D increases from 5 µg for individuals through age 50 years to 10 µg for those ages 51 to 70 years, and to 15 µg for those over age 70 years (IOM, 1997). Because vitamin D is not widely distributed in the food supply (it occurs naturally in liver, fatty fish, and egg yolk, and is routinely added to fluid milk, dried skim milk powder, and margarine), it is easy to envision diets that would not provide vitamin D in amounts recommended for older adults. Special attention to intakes of this vitamin is thus warranted for individuals in this category, particularly because endogenous synthesis is less efficient with advancing age (MacLaughlin and Holick, 1985). Use of a supplement containing vitamin D could be considered, particularly by those living in northern latitudes or who rarely receive sun exposure and do not regularly drink milk.

It has been estimated that from 10 to 30 percent of individuals over the age of 50 have low levels of gastric acidity, resulting in insufficient release of vitamin B_{12} from the protein to which it is bound in foods, and thereby resulting in reduced absorption of the vitamin. For this reason it is recommended that adults over the age of 50 obtain most of their RDA for vitamin B_{12} from synthetic sources (either in a supplement or in fortified foods) (IOM, 1998a).

LIFESTYLE FACTORS THAT AFFECT REQUIREMENTS

Alcohol Abuse

Alcoholism or alcohol abuse is associated with reduced food and nutrient intakes and a greater frequency of nutrient deficiencies, especially thiamin, niacin, vitamin B_6, and folate (IOM, 1998a). Chronic, excessive alcohol intake results in damaging physiological effects that may affect absorption, plasma concentrations, metabolism, and excretion of nutrients such as vitamin B_6 and folate. Specific nutrient requirements have not been established in relation to levels of alcohol consumption.

The importance of assuring adequate intakes of micronutrients in situations of alcohol abuse is emphasized by the greater frequency of nutrient deficiencies in alcoholics, an example of which is the irreversible consequences of the Wernicke-Korsakoff syndrome of severe thiamin deficiency. For uncontrolled alcoholics who are unable to correct their poor food intake habits, a nutrient supplement may be helpful in meeting their requirements for micronutrients.

Cigarette Smoking

Although blood folate concentrations have been reported to be lower in smokers than in nonsmokers (IOM, 1998a), data suggest that a low intake (Subar et al., 1990) rather than an increased requirement may account for the poorer folate status of smokers. In contrast, there is substantial evidence that smoking increases oxidative stress and metabolic turnover of vitamin C, thus recommended intakes of vitamin C are increased by 35 mg/day for smokers (IOM, 2000b).

DIETARY PLANNING FOR PEOPLE WHO ARE ILL

Just as is the case with healthy persons, planning diets for those who are ill first involves setting nutrient goals that are appropriate for their health status and nutrient needs. The Recommended Dietary Allowance (RDA), the Adequate Intake (AI), and the Tolerable Upper Intake Level (UL) are appropriate Dietary Reference Intakes (DRIs) for dietary planning for healthy individuals. However, some individuals who are ill have conditions that affect the

absorption, storage, metabolism, or excretion of one or more nutrients and, as a result, the DRIs for these nutrients must be modified
to take these disease-related factors into account. This section
describes a general approach for using the DRIs in these situations.
Once appropriate therapeutic goals are determined, they too must
be converted into a diet that the individual can acquire, afford, and
will eat.

Most diseases and conditions alter needs for only a few nutrients,
with other nutrient needs remaining similar to those of healthy
persons. In clinical practice it is usually assumed that unless there is
a specific deviation of a nutrient known to be associated with the
disease or condition, the individual is "healthy" with regard to that
nutrient and the RDAs or AIs are reasonable goals for individual
planning. Thus, the intake recommendation that is appropriate for
the individual's gender, age, level of physical activity, and physiological state (e.g., pregnancy, lactation) would apply.

Government agencies or other organizations frequently specify
that diets fed to patients or to institutionalized populations meet
previously established RDA or Recommended Nutrient Intake
(RNI) levels. The approaches described in this report to plan diets
for a low risk of inadequate nutrient intakes for groups and individuals would apply in these situations. For example, patients who are
not at nutritional risk, who do not require a nutrition intervention,
or who receive a regular diet, can be treated as a group unless their
nutritional status changes. Individual patients with specific nutrition therapy plans can have their dietary intakes planned initially
using the RDAs or AIs with appropriate modifications made for
their specific conditions by a trained health care professional or
dietitian.

After the appropriate nutrient goals for the individual who is ill
have been determined, these goals must then be converted into a
dietary pattern that the individual will consume. Therapeutic dietary
planning relies upon specialized food guidance and menu planning
systems specific to the various disease states that affect nutrient
needs. The DRIs will be useful in the development of diet manuals
for people with special health care needs. Parenterally-fed patients
require special forms of nutrients, and needs must be adjusted since
bioavailability factors are not applicable and absorptive losses do
not occur. Thus, the DRIs cannot be used directly to plan parenteral
intakes.

As an example, a uremic patient who has end-stage renal disease
might be placed on a very low protein diet to decrease blood urea
nitrogen and other biochemical indices of uremia and to provide

symptomatic relief. The diet might also be modified to restrict sodium and phosphorus. However, the RDA or AI would be used for other nutrients not known to be affected by the disease process.

The DRIs are formulated to meet the needs of the vast majority of the healthy population within specified life stage and gender groups. However, when the absorption, metabolism, or excretion of a nutrient is known to be altered by a specific illness or disease process, the DRIs can also be used as the base for developing therapeutic diets.

7
Implications and Recommendations

While developing the guidance for use of the Dietary Reference Intakes (DRIs) in planning diets for groups and individuals, several crucial areas have been identified for which data and techniques do not exist or for which additional knowledge is needed. This chapter synthesizes and prioritizes these needs. Research recommendations to improve the uses of the DRIs as applied to dietary assessment have been delineated (IOM, 2000a). As part of a necessary cycle of assessment, planning, implementation, and reassessment, a number of the research recommendations proposed for dietary assessment apply to dietary planning as well. These recommendations, which address issues such as the need to improve estimates of nutrient requirements and the quality of dietary intake data, are reiterated here. The recommendations in this chapter have been prioritized, and those presented under the first heading should be given the highest priority for research and development funding.

DIETARY PLANNING FOR GROUPS

Pilot test the proposed approach to planning for a low group prevalence of inadequacy.

The approach to group planning proposed in this report focuses on planning for intakes rather than meals offered or served and on the distribution of usual intakes rather than on mean intake. This approach aims to achieve a low prevalence of inadequate and excessive intakes of nutrients. However for some nutrients, achieving a low prevalence of inadequacy may require a considerable repositioning of the usual nutrient intake distribution, thus targeting a higher median intake than may have been customary when previous planning activities focused on the Recommended Dietary Allowance. Before large-scale implementation of such changes, practical pilot testing of this approach will be useful to assess whether a low prevalence of inadequacy can be achieved while meeting other important goals (e.g., avoiding excessive consumption of energy, maintaining nutrient intakes below the Tolerable Upper Intake Level [UL], and avoiding unnecessary food waste).

Determine how different nutrition interventions affect intake distributions.

It cannot be assumed that an intervention designed to increase the intake of a nutrient will result in a simple upward shift in nutrient intakes without changing the shape of the intake distribution or the between-person variation in usual nutrient intake. Different types of nutritional interventions may have very different effects on both the magnitude and shape of the intake distribution. A nearly complete distribution shift may be possible with interventions involving mandatory fortification of whole diets that have limited variety, such as emergency relief rations, or diets with a limited number of widely consumed staple foods in economically depressed areas of the world.

Successful government-sponsored fortification of varied diets, as is the case in the United States and Canada, depends on an appropriate selection of food vehicles that are similarly consumed by most people. Other nutritional interventions, based on supplementation recommendations, industry-initiated fortification of specific foods, increased food choices, or nutrition education approaches, have less predictable effects on the nutrient intake distribution. Some interventions may move the median intake while expanding the range and variation, resulting in little improvement or movement up or down at the extreme tails of the distribution. It is also possible that targeted interventions may affect primarily individuals in the tail of a distribution, thus changing the shape and benefiting those in greatest need of dietary improvement. Examination and publication of intake distributions before and after an intervention, with a systematic collection of this type of data, would allow a more informed selection of methods for planning a dietary intervention.

Determine the intake distributions of specific population groups.

Methods have been outlined in this report to estimate the distribution of usual intakes in a group and apply this estimate to position or target the distribution of usual intakes so that there is a low prevalence of dietary inadequacy or excess. Data on dietary intakes may be available for large groups, either from national population surveys or surveys of large groups (e.g., participants in the National School Lunch Program; the Supplemental Nutrition Program for Women, Infants, and Children; or specific branches of the military). However, often such information has not been reported in a manner that facilitates the estimation of variation in the usual intake of individuals. Information is generally minimal or lacking on the nutrient intake distributions of other groups such as children in different daycare settings, hospitalized patients, or residential long-term care homes or other institutional settings (with or without selective menus). For smaller settings where the on-site assessment of intake distributions may not be practical, planning for a low prevalence of inadequate intakes can be facilitated by descriptive data on the size and shape of intake distributions associated with similar settings. In addition, there is a paucity of population-level dietary intake data in Canada and on some underserved subgroups in the United States (e.g., Native Americans on reservations or inner city populations).

Conduct further research on the relationship between foods offered and nutrient intake in the context of group planning.

Although the framework for group planning focuses on the distribution of nutrient intakes as the ultimate goal, planners generally can control only what is offered and served to individuals in the group. More work is needed to provide guidance to planners on how food and nutrient offerings relate to food and nutrient intakes in various populations and how the relationship between offering and intake varies according to planning contexts.

Develop and evaluate dietary planning strategies for heterogeneous groups, including a nutrient-density approach to dietary planning.

Groups may be heterogeneous in ways (e.g., life stage and gender) that result in multiple requirement levels within the same group. The nutrient density approach is suggested here as a method to plan diets to achieve adequate amounts of nutrients for all group members based on those with the highest requirements. This approach involves planning for a minimum nutrient density in proportion to the energy content of the diet. Research is needed to determine the practical usefulness of planning for a target nutrient density, to determine if the applicability of the nutrient density approach is limited to situations with predetermined food allocations or restricted food choices (e.g., emergency relief rations), and to determine if this approach would be practical in situations offering a wide variety of food choices where the nutrient density is more dependent on food selection than on total food access to meet energy needs.

For situations in which nutrient density approaches are deemed useful, further development of data and methods is needed to estimate the median and distribution associated with nutrient requirements when expressed as a proportion of energy, either by statistical derivation from the present Estimated Average Requirements (EARs), or as a goal for future revisions of the Dietary Reference Intakes.

Further research is also necessary to determine how intake distributions for all nutrients are affected when plans for heterogeneous groups involve targeting the aggregate or average requirement of specific nutrients for all individuals within a group versus targeting the maximum individual requirement for the whole group. Criteria are needed to determine when to apply each of these approaches based upon current knowledge used to derive the EARs and ULs, studies of intake distributions, and the effects of interventions (see the analysis of folate intake distributions by Lewis and colleagues [1999]). These criteria should consider the impact of such goal setting on the food supply and resulting distribution of intakes.

RESEARCH TO IMPROVE THE QUALITY OF DIETARY INTAKE DATA

As discussed in the preceding chapters, planning diets, at either the individual or group level, involves setting goals for what nutrient intakes should be. Thus, in order to plan effectively, high-quality data are needed on dietary intake of nutrients.

Much has been written about ways to improve the quality of the intake data on which assessments are based (IOM, 2000a); some of the topics are revisited here along with specific areas in which research is still needed.

Important advances to improve the application of human nutrient requirement estimates have been made with the further development and refinement of statistical procedures to reduce, if not eliminate, the distorting effect of random error in dietary data (Nusser et al., 1996). The remaining issue of paramount importance in dietary data collection and analysis is the presence and true extent of bias (such as under- or overreporting of food intake) and the accuracy of food composition databases.

Research is needed to develop and validate statistical procedures to identify and correct for both under- and overreporting in self-reported intake data for energy and other nutrients.

This is a relatively unexplored field. Methods for directly estimating bias regarding energy intake have been developed and used to demonstrate that the problem is serious. While the underreporting of energy has now been well documented, it is unclear how this affects the accuracy of self-reported nutrient intakes. Research into this question has been limited by the absence of reference biomarkers of intake for many nutrients. Efforts have begun in the management of bias during data analysis, but these are far from satisfactory at present. Unfortunately, the methods available to reduce bias caused by energy underreporting do not provide an appropriate correction of underreporting for dietary intake data to be used in assessment and planning applications of the Dietary Reference Intakes (DRIs). The handling of bias is a high-priority area of research awaiting new initiatives and innovative approaches.

Better ways to quantify the intake of supplements are needed.

Methods for collecting accurate supplement intake data have not been widely investigated. For the Third National Health and Nutrition Examination Survey, different instruments were used to collect food intake data and supplement intake data, and the correct methodology for combining these data is uncertain. Furthermore, the intake distribution from supplements usually cannot be adjusted because the data do not permit the estimation of the day-to-day variability in supplement intake. Plans for the Fourth National Health and Nutrition Examination Survey attempt to address some of these issues. Despite the difficulties in maintaining a supplement composition database for the rapidly changing market, investigation of better methods of quantifying supplement intakes is a high-priority research area.

Food composition databases need to be updated to include the forms and units that are specified by DRIs.

Analysis of various forms of certain nutrients (e.g., α- versus γ-tocopherol) may be required. The DRI recommendations also imply that databases need to separate nutrients inherent in foods from those provided by fortification, particularly when intakes are compared with the Tolerable Upper Intake Level for nutrients (e.g., niacin). It has been suggested (IOM, 1998a, 2000b) that food composition databases report nutrients by weight and by equivalents to allow for rapid updates when more is known about bioavailability. Thus, it may also be necessary to change the units of measurement (e.g., dietary folate equivalents, as suggested for folate [IOM, 1998a]; the milligrams of α-tocopherol, suggested for vitamin E in place of α-tocopherol equivalents [IOM, 2000b], and new biological conversion rates for β-carotene to vitamin A as suggested for retinol activity equivalents in place of retinol equivalents [IOM, 2001]).

GUIDANCE FOR DIETARY PLANNING

Review and, where necessary, revise existing food guides.

Changes in recommended intakes of various nutrients, combined with rapid changes in the amount and number of nutrients and types of foods that are fortified (particularly in the United States), necessitate review of existing food guides and continuation of the periodic review of dietary guidance such as the Dietary Guidelines for Americans and Canada's Guidelines for Healthy Eating.

Develop technical tools for the professional.

There is a need to develop analytical tools that support implementation of recommendations for using the Dietary Reference Intakes (DRIs) for professional dietary assessment and planning, as well as for general guidelines for professionals to evaluate such tools. Industry and academia should explore development and production of accurate and convenient tools, expanding on the availability and use of sophisticated hand-held calculators and computers and easy Internet access to a spectrum of data and software.

Communicate with and educate nutrition professionals.

For full implementation and use of the DRIs, communication

strategies are needed to effectively educate nutrition professionals on how the DRI recommendations can be practically and effectively applied. The DRIs are more complex than past efforts (NRC, 1989; Health Canada, 1990b) and draw more and more from the realms of the basic sciences and mathematics. There is a need to formally examine how to best integrate this information into the education of nutrition professionals.

Assess application of the DRIs for food and supplement labeling.

The DRIs provide updated nutrient intake recommendations with scientific justification and extensive documentation. For some nutrients (e.g., folate and vitamin B_{12}), the need to evaluate appropriate labeling information in both the United States and Canada is recognized to convey the recommendation for synthetic sources. Developing and testing a labeling format that conveys the meaning and use of the Tolerable Upper Intake Level may be especially helpful to consumers.

Develop and evaluate food guides for group planning.

Planning for groups to have a low prevalence of inadequate dietary intakes involves methods different from those used in planning for a low risk of dietary inadequacy for individuals. However, in both cases, the emphasis should be on food sources of nutrients. In the United States food-based menu planning guides have long been part of specifications for professionals to use in planning the food offered in various nutrition programs such as the National School Lunch Program. Convenient-to-use, food-based guidelines for menu planning for specific groups should be developed to assist professionals in planning for a low group prevalence of inadequate or excessive intakes. As with the pilot testing of group planning methodologies already mentioned, such guides will need to be evaluated.

RESEARCH TO IMPROVE ESTIMATES OF NUTRIENT REQUIREMENTS

Even for nutrients for which an Estimated Average Requirement (EAR) is available, requirement data on which the EAR is based are typically scarce and usually only for adults. Such EARs and Recommended Dietary Allowances (RDAs) are often based on just a few experiments or studies with very small sample sizes, and therefore considerable uncertainty exists about the true median and standard deviation of the distribution of requirements within a group. Given the importance of median and distribution of requirements in both assessment and planning, additional carefully conducted research is needed in this area to accomplish the tasks discussed below.

Improve existing estimates of the EAR and RDA.

There is need to both improve the database of controlled experimental studies relevant to the EAR, as well as to broaden the approach to estimating requirements. Congruence of evidence should be expected from different sources, including population based and clinical investigations as well as experimental and factorial approaches, before being truly confident in an EAR.

Provide better information on requirements so it becomes possible to establish an EAR (and thus an RDA) for nutrients that currently have Adequate Intakes (AIs).

Research that allows replacement of the AIs with EARs for age groups older than infants will allow for additional applications. As discussed in earlier chapters, EARs present more possibilities for assessing individual and group prevalence of inadequacy and especially for planning for low group prevalence of inadequacy.

Improve estimates of the distribution of requirements so that the appropriate method for assessing the prevalence of inadequacy for groups can be determined (cut-point method versus probability approach).

Research in this area is also needed to enable more accurate applications of the Dietary Reference Intakes to specific individuals and populations. Adjustment factors for considerations such as body size, physical activity, and intakes of energy and other nutrients may be appropriate but are often unknown. Studies to evaluate nutrient requirements or adverse effects should provide individual data where possible to allow estimation of their distributions.

Identify factors that can alter the upper intake levels that can be tolerated biologically.

Establishment of Tolerable Upper Intake Levels (ULs) provides an opportunity to evaluate the risk of adverse effects for individuals and populations and is an extremely important step forward in assessing nutrient intakes. Research to allow ULs to be set for all nutrients should be undertaken in carefully controlled settings. In addition, information on the distribution of adverse effects via dose–response data (e.g., risk curves) would allow greatly expanded applications of the UL, particularly for population groups. More information is needed on ways to identify and conceptualize the risk of exceeding the UL.

8

References

ACC/SCN (Administrative Committee on Coordination/Sub-Committee on Nutrition). 2000. *Fourth Report on The World Nutrition Situation.* Geneva: ACC/SCN in collaboration with IFPRI. Pp. 27–29.

Aickin M, Ritenbaugh C. 1991. Estimation of the true distribution of vitamin A intake by the unmixing algorithm. *Commun Stat Sim* 20:255–280.

ARS (Agriculture Research Service). 1998. *Continuing Survey of Food Intakes by Individuals (CSFII) 1994–96, 1998.* CD-ROM. Beltsville, MD: ARS.

Bandini LG, Schoeller DA, Cry HN, Dietz WH. 1990. Validity of reported energy intake in obese and nonobese adolescents. *Am J Clin Nutr* 52:421–425.

Beaton GH. 1994. Criteria of an adequate diet. In: Shils ME, Olson JA, Shike M, eds. *Modern Nutrition in Health and Disease,* 8th ed. Philadelphia: Lea & Febiger. Pp. 1491–1505.

Beaton GH, Milner J, McGuire V, Feather TE, Little JA. 1983. Source of variance in 24-hour dietary recall data: Implications for nutrition study design and interpretation. Carbohydrate sources, vitamins, and minerals. *Am J Clin Nutr* 37:986–995.

Beaton GH, Burema J, Ritenbaugh C. 1997. Errors in interpretation of dietary assessments. *Am J Clin Nutr* 65:1100S–1107S.

Becker W, Welten D. 2001. Under-reporting in dietary surveys—implications for development of food-based dietary guidelines. *Public Health Nutr* 4:683–687.

Becker W, Foley S, Shelley E, Gibney M. 1999. Energy under-reporting in Swedish and Irish dietary surveys: Implications for food-based dietary guidelines. *Br J Nutr* 81:S127–S131.

Berner LA, Clydesdale FM, Douglass JS. 2001. Fortification contributed greatly to vitamin and mineral intakes in the United States, 1989–1991. *J Nutr* 131:2177–2183.

Black AE, Cole TJ. 2001. Biased over- or under-reporting is characteristic of individuals whether over time or by different assessment methods. *J Am Diet Assoc* 101:70–80.

Black AE, Goldberg GR, Jebb SA, Livingstone MBE, Cole TJ, Prentice AM. 1991. Critical evaluation of energy intake data using fundamental principles of energy physiology: 2. Evaluating the results of published surveys. *Eur J Clin Nutr* 45:583–599.

Black AE, Prentice AM, Goldberg GR, Jebb SA, Bingham SA, Livingstone MB, Conward WA. 1993. Measurements of total energy expenditure provide insights into the validity of dietary measurements of energy intake. *J Am Diet Assoc* 93:572–579.

Briefel RR, Sempos CT, McDowell MA, Chien S, Alaimo K. 1997. Dietary methods research in the Third National Health and Nutrition Examination Survey: Underreporting of energy intake. *Am J Clin Nutr* 65:1203S–1209S.

Burghardt JA, Gordon AR, Fraker TM. 1995. Meals offered in the national school lunch program and the school breakfast program. *Am J Clin Nutr* 61:187S–198S.

CDC/NCHS (Centers for Disease Control and Prevention/National Center for Health Statistics). 2000. *2000 CDC Growth Charts*. Online. Available at http://www.cdc.gov/growthcharts/. Accessed December 3, 2002.

CFIA (Canadian Food Inspection Agency). 1996. *Guide to Food Labelling and Advertising*. Online. Available at http://www.inspection.gc.ca/english/bureau/labeti/guide/guidee.shtml. Accessed December 3, 2002.

COMA (Committee on Medical Aspects of Food Policy). 1991. *Dietary Reference Values for Food Energy and Nutrients for the United Kingdom*. Report on Health and Social Subjects, No. 41. London: Her Majesty's Stationary Office.

Consumer and Corporate Affairs Canada. 1988. *Guide for Food Manufacturers and Advertisers*. Ottawa: Consumer Products Branch, Bureau of Consumer Affairs.

Demirjian A. 1980. *Anthropometry Report. Height, Weight, and Body Dimensions: A Report from Nutrition Canada*. Ottawa: Minister of National Health and Welfare, Health and Promotion Directorate, Health Services and Promotion Branch.

Devaney BL, Gordon AR, Burghardt JA. 1995. Dietary intakes of students. *Am J Clin Nutr* 61:205S–221S.

FAO/WHO (Food and Agriculture Organization/World Health Organization). 1970. *Requirements of Ascorbic Acid, Vitamin D, Vitamin B_{12}, Folate, and Iron. Report of a Joint FAO/WHO Expert Group*. WHO Technical Report Series No. 452. Geneva: WHO.

FAO/WHO. 1988. *Requirements of Vitamin A, Iron, Folate, and Vitamin B_{12}. Report of a Joint FAO/WHO Expert Consultation*. FAO Food and Nutrition Series No. 23. Rome: FAO.

FAO/WHO/UNU (United Nations University). 1985. *Energy and Protein Requirements. Report of a Joint FAO/WHO/UNU Expert Consultation*. Technical Report Series No. 724. Geneva: WHO.

FDA (U.S. Food and Drug Administration). 1999. *The Food Label*. FDA Backgrounder. May 1999. Online. Center for Food Safety and Applied Nutrition. Available at http://www.cfsan.fda.gov/~dms/fdnewlab.html. Accessed November 18, 2002.

FDA. 2000. *Guidance on How to Understand and Use the Nutrition Facts Panel on Food Labels*. Online. Center for Food Safety and Applied Nutrition. Available at http://www.cfsan.fda.gov/~dms/foodlab.html. Accessed May 16, 2002.

Fox MK, Crepinsek MK, Connor P, Battaglia M. 2001. *School Nutrition Dietary Assessment Study: II. Final Report*. Washington, DC: U.S. Department of Agriculture, Food and Nutrition Service.

Gentle JE. 1998. *Random Number Generation and Monte Carlo Methods*. New York: Springer-Verlag.

Goldberg GR, Black AE, Jebb SA, Cole TJ, Murgatroyd PR, Conward WA, Prentice AM. 1991. Critical evaluation of energy intake data using fundamental principles of energy physiology: 1. Derivation of cut-off limits to identify under-recording. *Eur J Clin Nutr* 45:569–581.

Goris AHC, Westerterp-Plantenga MS, Westerterp KR. 2000. Undereating and underrecording of habitual food intake in obese men: Selective underreporting of fat intake. *Am J Clin Nutr* 71:130–134.

Goyeneche JJ, Carriquiry A, Fuller WA. 1997. Estimating bivariate usual intake distributions. *ASA Proceedings of the Biometrics Section*. Alexandria, VA: American Statistical Association.

Guenther PM, Kott PS, Carriquiry AL. 1997. Development of an approach for estimating usual nutrient intake distributions at the population level. *J Nutr* 127:1106–1112.

Health Canada. 1990a. *Action Towards Healthy Eating. Canada's Guidelines for Healthy Eating and Recommended Strategies for Implementation*. The Report of the Communications/Implementation Committee. Ottawa: Public Works and Government Service Canada.

Health Canada. 1990b. *Nutrition Recommendations*. The Report of the Scientific Review Committee 1990. Ottawa: Canadian Government Publishing Centre.

Health Canada. 1991. *Canada's Food Guide to Healthy Eating*. Ottawa: Minister of Supply and Services.

Health Canada. 1997. *Using the Food Guide*. Ottawa: Public Works and Government Service Canada.

Health Canada. 1998. *Handbook for Canada's Physical Activity Guide to Healthy Active Living*. Ottawa: Health Canada and the Canadian Society for Exercise Physiology.

Health Canada. 1999. *The Addition of Vitamins and Minerals to Foods: Proposed Policy Recommendations*. Ottawa: Bureau of Nutritional Sciences, Food Directorate, Health Protection Branch.

Health Canada. 2002. *Nutrition Labels*. Online. Available at http://www.hc-sc.gc.ca/hppb/nutrition/labels/e_before.html. Accessed November 27, 2002.

Herman-Giddens ME, Slora EJ, Wasserman RC, Bourdony CJ, Bhapkar MV, Koch GG, Hasemeier CM. 1997. Secondary sexual characteristics and menses in young girls seen in office practice: A study from the Pediatric Research in Office Settings Network. *Pediatrics* 99:505–512.

HHS (U.S. Department of Health and Human Services). 1996. *Physical Activity and Health: A Report of the Surgeon General*. Atlanta: Centers for Disease Control and Prevention, National Center for Chronic Disease Prevention and Health Promotion.

Hoffmann K, Boeing H, Dufour A, Volatier JL, Telman J, Virtanen M, Becker S, DeHenauw S. 2002. Estimating the distribution of usual dietary intake by short-term measures. *Eur J Clin Nutr* 56:S53–S62.

Hunt JR, Roughead ZK. 1999. Nonheme-iron absorption, fecal ferritin excretion, and blood indexes of iron status in women consuming controlled lactoovo-vegetarian diets for 8 wk. *Am J Clin Nutr* 69:944–952.

Hunt JR, Matthys LA, Johnson LK. 1998. Zinc absorption, mineral balance, and blood lipids in women consuming controlled lactoovovegetarian and omnivorous diets for 8 wk. *Am J Clin Nutr* 67:421–430.

IOM (Institute of Medicine). 1990. *Nutrition During Pregnancy: Part I: Weight Gain, Part II: Nutrient Supplements*. Washington, DC: National Academy Press.

IOM. 1992. *Nutrition During Pregnancy and Lactation: An Implementation Guide*. Washington, DC: National Academy Press.

IOM. 1994. *How Should the Recommended Dietary Allowances Be Revised?* Washington, DC: National Academy Press.

IOM. 1995. *Estimated Mean per Capita Energy Requirements for Planning Emergency Food Aid Rations.* Washington, DC: National Academy Press.

IOM. 1997. *Dietary Reference Intakes for Calcium, Phosphorus, Magnesium, Vitamin D, and Fluoride.* Washington, DC: National Academy Press.

IOM. 1998a. *Dietary Reference Intakes for Thiamin, Riboflavin, Niacin, Vitamin B$_6$, Folate, Vitamin B$_{12}$, Pantothenic Acid, Biotin, and Choline.* Washington, DC: National Academy Press.

IOM. 1998b. *Prevention of Micronutrient Deficiencies: Tools for Policymakers and Public Health Workers.* Washington, DC: National Academy Press.

IOM. 1999. *Dietary Reference Intakes: A Risk Assessment Model for Establishing Upper Intake Levels for Nutrients.* Washington, DC: National Academy Press.

IOM. 2000a. *Dietary Reference Intakes: Applications in Dietary Assessment.* Washington, DC: National Academy Press.

IOM. 2000b. *Dietary Reference Intakes for Vitamin C, Vitamin E, Selenium, and Carotenoids.* Washington, DC: National Academy Press.

IOM. 2001. *Dietary Reference Intakes for Vitamin A, Vitamin K, Arsenic, Boron, Chromium, Copper, Iodine, Iron, Manganese, Molybdenum, Nickel, Silicon, Vanadium, and Zinc.* Washington, DC: National Academy Press.

IOM. 2002a. *Dietary Reference Intakes for Energy, Carbohydrate, Fiber, Fat, Fatty Acids, Cholesterol, Protein, and Amino Acids.* Washington, DC: National Academy Press.

IOM. 2002b. *High-Energy, Nutrient-Dense Emergency Relief Food Product.* Washington, DC: National Academy Press.

Jacques PF, Bostom AG, Williams RR, Ellison RC, Eckfeldt JH, Rosenberg IH, Selhub J, Rozen R. 1996. Relation between folate status, a common mutation in methylenetetrahydrofolate reductase, and plasma homocysteine concentrations. *Circulation* 93:7–9.

Johansson L, Solvoll K, Aa Bjorneboe G-E, Drevon CA. 1998. Under- and over-reporting of energy intake related to weight status and lifestyle in a nationwide sample. *Am J Clin Nutr* 68:266–274.

Johnson RK, Soultanakis RP, Matthews DE. 1998. Literacy and body fatness are associated with underreporting of energy intake in US low-income women using the multiple-pass 24-hour recall: A doubly labeled water study. *J Am Diet Assoc* 98:1136–1140.

Kaczkowski CH, Jones PJH, Feng J, Bayley HS. 2000. Four-day multimedia diet records underestimate energy needs in middle-aged and elderly women as determined by doubly-labeled water. *J Nutr* 130:802–805.

Krebs-Smith SM, Graubard BI, Kahle LL, Subar AF, Cleveland LE, Ballard-Barbash R. 2000. Low energy reporters vs. others: A comparison of reported food intakes. *Eur J Clin Nutr* 54:281–287.

Kuczmarski MF, Kuczmarski RJ, Najjar M. 2001. Effects of age on validity of self-reported height, weight, and body mass index: Findings from the Third National Health and Nutrition Examination Survey, 1988–1994. *J Am Diet Assoc* 101:28–34.

Kuczmarski RJ, Ogden CL, Grummer-Strawn LM, Flegal KM, Guo SS, Wei R, Mei Z, Curtin LR, Roche AF, Johnson CL. 2000. CDC growth charts: United States. *Advance Data from Vital and Health Statistics* 314:1–28.

Ladizesky M, Lu Z, Oliveri B, San Roman N, Diaz S, Holick MF, Mautalen C. 1995. Solar ultraviolet B radiation and photoproduction of vitamin D$_3$ in central and southern areas of Argentina. *J Bone Miner Res* 10:545–549.

Larsson CL, Westerterp KR, Johansson GK. 2002. Validity of reported energy expenditure and energy and protein intakes in Swedish adolescent vegans and omnivores. *Am J Clin Nutr* 75:268–274.

Lewis CJ, Crane NT, Wilson DB, Yetley EA. 1999. Estimated folate intakes: Data updated to reflect food fortification, increased bioavailability, and dietary supplement use. *Am J Clin Nutr* 70:198–207.

MacLaughlin J, Holick MF. 1985. Aging decreases the capacity of human skin to produce vitamin D. *J Clin Invest* 76:1536–1538.

Martin LJ, Su W, Jones PJ, Lockwood GA, Tritchler DL, Boyd NF. 1996. Comparison of energy intakes determined by food records and doubly labeled water in women participating in a dietary-intervention trial. *Am J Clin Nutr* 63:483–490.

Mertz W, Tsui JC, Judd JT, Reiser S, Hallfrisch J, Morris ER, Steele PD, Lashley E. 1991. What are people really eating? The relation between energy intake derived from estimated diet records and intake determined to maintain body weight. *Am J Clin Nutr* 54:291–295.

Mertz W, Abernathy CO, Olin SS. 1994. *Risk Assessment of Essential Elements*. Washington, DC: ILSI Press.

Messina VK, Burke KI. 1997. Position of the American Dietetic Association: Vegetarian diets. *J Am Diet Assoc* 97:1317–1321.

Monsen ER, Hallberg L, Layrisse M, Hegsted DM, Cook JD, Mertz W, Finch CA. 1978. Estimation of available dietary iron. *Am J Clin Nutr* 31:134–141.

Northwest Territories Aboriginal Head Start Program. 2002. *N.W.T. Food Guide*. Online. Available at www.nwtheadstart.org/comp_nutrition_food_guide.htm. Accessed August 16, 2002.

NRC (National Research Council). 1968. *Recommended Dietary Allowances,* 7th ed. Washington, DC: National Academy Press.

NRC. 1986. *Nutrient Adequacy: Assessment Using Food Consumption Surveys*. Washington, DC: National Academy Press.

NRC. 1989. *Recommended Dietary Allowances,* 10th ed. Washington, DC: National Academy Press.

Nusser SM, Carriquiry AL, Dodd KW, Fuller WA. 1996. A semiparametric transformation approach to estimating usual daily intake distributions. *J Am Stat Assoc* 91:1440–1449.

PCRM (Physicians Committee for Responsible Medicine). 1997. The origin of U.S. Dietary Guidelines. Online. *Good Medicine*. Available at http://www.pcrm.org/magazine/GM97Autumn/GM97Autumn2.html. Accessed November 27, 2002.

Pett LB, Ogilvie GH. 1956. The Canadian Weight-Height Survey. *Hum Biol* 28:177–188.

Prentice AM, Black AE, Coward WA, Davies HL, Goldberg GR, Murgatroyd PR, Ashford J, Sawyer M, Whitehead RG. 1986. High levels of energy expenditure in obese women. *Br Med J* 292:983–987.

Saint L, Maggiore P, Hartmann PE. 1986. Yield and nutrient content of milk in eight women breast-feeding twins and one woman breast-feeding triplets. *Br J Nutr* 56:49–58.

Sawaya AL, Tucker K, Tsay R, Willett W, Saltzman E, Dallal GE, Roberts SB. 1996. Evaluation of four methods for determining energy intake in young and older women: Comparison with doubly labeled water measurements of total energy expenditure. *Am J Clin Nutr* 63:491–499.

Shaw A, Fulton L, Davis C, Hogbin M. 1996. *Using the Food Guide Pyramid: A Resource for Nutrition Education*. Washington, DC: U.S. Department of Agriculture, Food, Nutrition and Consumer Services, Center for Nutrition Policy and Promotion.

Sichert-Hellert W, Kersting M, Schöh G. 1999. Consumption of fortified foods between 1985 and 1996 in 2- to 14-year-old German children and adolescents. *Int J Food Sci Nutr* 50:65–72.

Stallone DD, Brunner EJ, Bingham SA, Marmot MG. 1997. Dietary assessment in Whitehall II: The influence of reporting bias on apparent socioeconomic variation in nutrient intakes. *Eur J Clin Nutr* 51:815–825.

Steel RGD, Torrie JH, Dickey DA. 1997. *Principles and Procedures of Statistics. A Biometrical Approach*, 3rd ed. Boston: WCB McGraw-Hill. P. 612.

Subar AF, Harlan LC, Mattson ME. 1990. Food and nutrient intake differences between smokers and non-smokers in the US. *Am J Public Health* 80:1323–1329.

Tarasuk VS, Beaton GH. 1999. Women's dietary intakes in the context of household food insecurity. *J Nutr* 129:672–679.

Tomoyasu NJ, Toth MJ, Poehlman ET. 1999. Misreporting of total energy intake in older men and women. *J Am Geriatr Soc* 47:710–715.

USDA (U.S. Department of Agriculture). 1992. *The Food Guide Pyramid.* Home and Garden Bulletin No. 252. Washington, DC: U.S. Government Printing Office.

USDA/ARS (Agricultural Research Service). 1997. *1994–96 Continuing Survey of Food Intakes by Individuals (CSFII 1994–96)*. Riverdale, MD: USDA.

USDA/HHS (U.S. Department of Health and Human Services). 1980. *Nutrition and Your Health: Dietary Guidelines for Americans.* Home and Garden Bulletin No. 232. Washington, DC: U.S. Government Printing Office.

USDA/HHS. 2000. *Nutrition and Your Health: Dietary Guidelines for Americans,* 5th ed. Home and Garden Bulletin No. 232. Washington, DC: U.S. Government Printing Office.

Welsh SO, Davis C, Shaw A. 1993. *USDA's Food Guide: Background and Development.* Miscellaneous Publication No. 1514. Hyattsville, MD: USDA.

Webb AR, Kline L, Holick MF. 1988. Influence of season and latitude on the cutaneous synthesis of vitamin D_3: Exposure to winter sunlight in Boston and Edmonton will not promote vitamin D_3 synthesis in human skin. *J Clin Endocrinol Metab* 67:373–378.

Whittaker P, Tufaro PR, Rader JL. 2001. Iron and folate in fortified cereals. *J Am Coll Nutr* 20:247–254.

Willett W, Stampfer MJ. 1986. Total energy intake: Implications for epidemiologic analyses. *Am J Epidemiol* 124:17–27.

A

Origin and Framework of the Development of Dietary Reference Intakes

This report is one of a series of publications resulting from the comprehensive effort being undertaken by the Food and Nutrition Board's (FNB) Standing Committee on the Scientific Evaluation of Dietary Reference Intakes (DRI Committee) and its panels and subcommittees.

ORIGIN

This initiative began in June 1993, when FNB organized a symposium and public hearing entitled, "Should the Recommended Dietary Allowances Be Revised?" Shortly thereafter, to continue its collaboration with the larger nutrition community on the future of the Recommended Dietary Allowances (RDAs), FNB took two major steps: (1) it prepared, published, and disseminated the concept paper, "How Should the Recommended Dietary Allowances Be Revised?" (IOM, 1994), which invited comments regarding the proposed concept, and (2) it held several symposia at nutrition-focused professional meetings to discuss FNB's tentative plans and to receive responses to the initial concept paper. Many aspects of the conceptual framework of the DRIs came from the United Kingdom's report, *Dietary Reference Values for Food Energy and Nutrients for the United Kingdom* (COMA, 1991).

The five general conclusions presented in FNB's 1994 concept paper were:

1. Sufficient new information has accumulated to support a reassessment of the RDAs.

2. Where sufficient data for efficacy and safety exist, reduction in the risk of chronic degenerative disease is a concept that should be included in the formulation of future recommendations.

3. Upper levels of intake should be established where data exist regarding risk of toxicity.

4. Components of food that may benefit health, although not meeting the traditional concept of a nutrient, should be reviewed, and if adequate data exist, reference intakes should be established.

5. Serious consideration must be given to developing a new format for presenting future recommendations.

Subsequent to the symposium and the release of the concept paper, FNB held workshops at which invited experts discussed many issues related to the development of nutrient-based reference values. (FNB and DRI Committee members have continued to provide updates and engage in discussions at professional meetings.) In addition, FNB gave attention to the international uses of the earlier RDAs and the expectation that the scientific review of nutrient requirements should be similar for comparable populations.

Concurrently, Health Canada and Canadian scientists were reviewing the need for revision of the *Recommended Nutrient Intakes* (RNIs) (Health Canada, 1990b). Consensus following a symposium for Canadian scientists, cosponsored by the Canadian National Institute of Nutrition and Health Canada in April 1995, was that the Canadian government should pursue the extent to which involvement with the developing FNB process would benefit both Canada and the United States in leading toward harmonization.

Based on extensive input and deliberations, FNB initiated action to provide a framework for the development and possible international harmonization of nutrient-based recommendations that would serve, where warranted, for all of North America. To this end, in December 1995, FNB began a close collaboration with the government of Canada and took action to establish the DRI Committee. It is hoped that representatives from Mexico will join in future deliberations.

THE CHARGE TO THE COMMITTEE

In 1995, the DRI Committee was appointed to oversee and conduct this project. It devised a plan involving the work of seven or more expert nutrient group panels and two overarching subcommittees (Figure A-1).

The Subcommittee on Interpretation and Uses of Dietary Reference Intakes (Uses Subcommittee), composed of experts in nutrition, dietetics, statistics, nutritional epidemiology, public health, economics, and consumer perspectives, was to (1) review the scientific literature regarding the uses of dietary reference standards and their applications, (2) provide guidance for the appropriate application of DRIs for specific purposes and identify inappropriate applications, (3) provide guidance for adjustments to be made for potential errors in dietary intake data and the assumptions regarding intake and requirement distributions, (4) provide specific guidance for use of DRI values for individual nutrients, and (5) identify research needed to improve the statistical underpinnings regarding quantitative applications of the DRIs for assessing and planning diets for individuals and for groups.

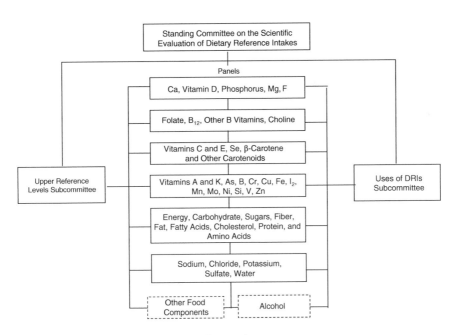

FIGURE A-1 Dietary Reference Intakes project structure.

This second report from the Uses Subcommittee examines the appropriate uses of each of the DRI values in *planning* nutrient intakes of groups and of individuals; an earlier report presented information on the appropriate uses of specific DRI values in *assessing* diets for groups and for individuals (IOM, 2000a). Each report presents the statistical underpinnings for the various uses of the DRI values and also indicates when specific uses are inappropriate. This report reflects the work of the DRI Committee, the Uses Subcommittee, and the Subcommittee on Upper Reference Levels of Nutrients.

ISSUES OF RELEVANCE FROM PAST DIETARY REFERENCE INTAKE REPORTS

Methodology to Develop Estimated Average Requirements and Recommended Dietary Allowances When Requirements for Nutrients Are Not Normally Distributed

For most of the nutrients for which Estimated Average Requirements (EARs) have been established, the required assumption of distribution of requirements is that of symmetry about the mean. In the case of iron, a nutrient of concern in many subgroups in the population in the United States, Canada, and other areas, requirements are known to follow a nonnormal distribution (IOM, 2001). Thus, a different method was needed to determine the intake of iron at which half of the individuals would be expected to be inadequate in the criterion used to establish adequacy (the EAR), and also to construct an intake level at which only a small percentage of the population would be inadequate (the RDA). Similar adjustments were made for dietary protein (IOM, 2002a).

If the requirement of a nutrient is not normally distributed but can be transformed to normality, its EAR and RDA can be estimated by transforming the data, calculating the 50th and 97.5th percentiles, and transforming these percentiles back into the original units. In this case, the difference between the EAR and the RDA cannot be used to obtain an estimate of the standard deviation or the coefficient of variation because skewing is usually present.

Where factorial modeling is used to estimate the distribution of requirements from the distributions of the individual components of requirement, as was done in the case of iron recommendations (IOM, 2001), it is necessary to add the individual distributions (convolutions). This is easy to do given that the average requirement is simply the sum of the averages of the individual component distributions, and a standard deviation of the combined distribution can be estimated by standard statistical techniques. The 97.5th percentile can then be estimated (for a further elaboration of this method, see Chapter 9 and Appendix I of *Dietary Reference Intakes for Vitamin A, Vitamin K, Arsenic, Boron, Chromium, Copper, Iodine, Iron, Manganese, Molybdenum, Nickel, Silicon, Vanadium, and Zinc* [IOM, 2001]).

If normality cannot be assumed for all of the components of requirement, then Monte Carlo simulation is used for the summation of the components. This approach models the distributions of the individual components and randomly assigns values to a large simulated population. The total requirement is then calculated for each individual and the median and the 97.5th percentile are calculated directly. As was the case for iron (IOM, 2001), the underlying joint distribution is approximated and a large number of individuals (100,000) are randomly generated. Information about the distribution of values for the requirement components is modeled on the basis of known physiology. Monte Carlo approaches may be used in the simulation of the distribution of components, or where large data sets exist for similar populations (data sets such as growth rates in infants), estimates of relative variability may be transferred to the component in the simulated population (Gentle, 1998). At each step the goal is to achieve distribution values for the component that not only reflect known physiology or known direct observations, but also can be transformed into a distribution that can be modeled and used in selecting random members to contribute to the final requirement distribution. When the final distribution representing the convolution of components has been derived, the median and 97.5th percentiles of the distribution can be directly estimated. It is recognized that in its simplest form, the Monte Carlo approach ignores possible correlation among components. In the case of iron, however, expected correlation is built into the modeling of requirement where components are linked to a common variable (e.g., growth rate) so that not all sources of correlation are neglected.

Life Stage Groups

Nutrient intake recommendations are expressed for 22 life stage groups, as listed in Table A-1 and described in more detail elsewhere (IOM, 1997). If data are too sparse to distinguish differences in requirements by life stage and gender, the analysis may be presented for a larger grouping. Differences are indicated by gender when warranted by the data.

TABLE A-1 The 22 Life Stage Groups for Which Dietary Reference Intakes (DRIs) are Given

Life Stage Groups

Infants	Males	Females	Pregnancy
0–6 mo	9–13 y	9–13 y	≤ 18 y
7–12 mo	14–18 y	14–18 y	19–30 y
	19–30 y	19–30 y	31–50 y
Children	31–50 y	31–50 y	
1–3 y	51–70 y	51–70 y	Lactation
4–8 y	> 70 y	> 70 y	≤ 18 y
			19–30 y
			31–50 y

NOTE: Differences in DRIs are indicated by gender when warranted by the data.

Reference Heights and Weights Used in Extrapolating Dietary Reference Intakes for Vitamins and Elements

The most up-to-date data providing heights and weights of individuals in the United States and Canada when the DRI process was initiated in 1995 were anthropometric data from the 1988–1994 Third National Health and Nutrition Examination Survey (NHANES III) in the United States, and older data from Canada. Reference values derived from the NHANES III data and used in previous reports are given in Table A-2. The earlier values were obtained as follows: the median heights for the life stage and gender groups through age 30 years were identified, and the median weights for these heights were based on reported median Body Mass Index (BMI) for the same individuals. Since there is no evidence that weight should change as adults age if activity is maintained, the reference weights for adults aged 19 through 30 years were applied to all adult age groups.

The most recent nationally representative data available for Canadians (from the 1970–1972 Nutrition Canada Survey [Demirjian, 1980]) were also reviewed. In general, median heights of children from 1 year of age in the United States were greater by 3 to 8 cm (1 to 2.5 in) than those of children of the same age in Canada measured two decades earlier (Demirjian, 1980). This difference could be partly explained by approximations necessary to compare the two data sets, but more likely by a continuation of the secular

TABLE A-2 Reference Heights and Weights for Children and Adults in the United States Used in the Vitamin and Element Dietary Reference Intake Reports[a] through 2001

Sex	Age	Median Body Mass Index (kg/m²)	Reference Height, cm (in)	Reference Weight[b] kg (lb)
Male, female	2–6 mo	—	64 (25)	7 (16)
	7–12 mo	—	72 (28)	9 (20)
	1–3 y	—	91 (36)	13 (29)
	4–8 y	15.8	118 (46)	22 (48)
Male	9–13 y	18.5	147 (58)	40 (88)
	14–18 y	21.3	174 (68)	64 (142)
	19–30 y	24.4	176 (69)	76 (166)
Female	9–13 y	18.3	148 (58)	40 (88)
	14–18 y	21.3	163 (64)	57 (125)
	19–30 y	22.8	163 (64)	61 (133)

[a] IOM (1997, 1998a, 2000b, 2001). Adapted from the Third National Health and Nutrition Examination Survey, 1988–1994.
[b] Calculated from body mass index and height for ages 4 through 8 years and older.

trend of increased heights for age noted in the Nutrition Canada Survey when it compared data from that survey with an earlier (1953) national Canadian survey (Pett and Ogilvie, 1956).

Similarly, median weights beyond age 1 year derived from the recent survey in the United States (NHANES III) were also greater than those obtained from the older Canadian survey (Demirjian, 1980). Differences were greatest during adolescence, ranging from 10 to 17 percent higher. The differences probably reflect the secular trend of earlier onset of puberty (Herman-Giddens et al., 1997), rather than differences in populations. Calculations of BMI for young adults (e.g., a median of 22.6 for Canadian women compared to 22.8 for U.S. women) resulted in similar values, thus indicating greater concordance between the two surveys by adulthood.

The reference weights used in the previous DRI reports (IOM, 1997, 1998a, 2000a, 2000b, 2001) were thus based on the most recent data set available from either country, with recognition that earlier surveys in Canada indicated shorter stature and lower weights during adolescence than did surveys in the United States.

New Reference Heights and Weights

As discussed earlier, when the DRI process was undertaken in 1994, the references heights and weights used were developed based on NHANES III data on BMI for children and young adults (IOM, 1997). Given the increasing prevalence of overweight and obesity in both adults and children (HHS, 1996), use of such population data is of concern. However, recent data providing heights and ideal BMIs for adults (Kuczmarski et al., 2000) and new growth charts for infants and children have allowed the development of new reference heights and weights (Table A-3) that should more closely approximate ideal weights based on low risk of chronic disease and adequate growth for children. These new values were used in the DRI report published in 2002 (IOM, 2002a) and will be used in subsequent DRI reports until they need to be revised based on new data or because of a conceptual need.

TABLE A-3 New Reference Heights and Weights for Children and Adults in the United States

Sex	Age	Previous Median Body Mass Index[a] (BMI) (kg/m^2)	New Median BMI[b] (kg/m^2)	New Median Reference Height[b] cm (in)	New Reference Weight[c] kg (lb)
Male, female	2–6 mo	—	—	62 (24)	6 (13)
	7–12 mo	—	—	71 (28)	9 (20)
	1–3 y	—	—	86 (34)	12 (27)
	4–8 y	15.8	15.3	115 (45)	20 (44)
Male	9–13 y	18.5	17.2	144 (57)	36 (79)
	14–18 y	21.3	20.5	174 (68)	61 (134)
	19–30 y	24.4	22.5	177 (70)	70 (154)
Female	9–13 y	18.3	17.4	144 (57)	37 (81)
	14–18 y	21.3	20.4	163 (64)	54 (119)
	19–30 y	22.8	21.5	163 (64)	57 (126)

[a] Taken from male and female median BMI and height-for-age data from the Third National Health and Nutrition Examination Survey (NHANES III), 1988–1994; used in earlier DRI reports (IOM 1997, 1998a, 2000b, 2001).
[b] Taken from new data on male and female median BMI and height-for-age data from the Centers for Disease Control and Prevention/National Center for Health Statistics Growth Charts (CDC/NCHS, 2000; Kuczmarski et al., 2000).
[c] Calculated from CDC/NCHS Growth Charts (CDC/NCHS, 2000; Kuczmarski et al., 2000), median BMI and median height for ages 4 through 19 years.

B

Food Guidance in the United States and Canada

FOOD GUIDES

The U.S. Food Guide Pyramid

Dietary guidance began in the early 1900s in the United States with the development of food guides that identified food groups and patterns for eating. In the 1940s, the food groups were identified as the Basic 7. By 1960, guidance was simplified into the basic four food groups. As nutrition science evolved, so did concern about some nutrients in excess (e.g., fats, saturated fat, cholesterol, sodium) and their relation to heart disease and cancer. These concerns led to the promulgation of the U.S. Dietary Goals in 1977 by the Senate Select Committee on Nutrition and Human Needs. The U.S. Department of Agriculture (USDA) responded by adding a fifth food group of fats, sweets, and alcohol at the bottom of the basic four, with the guidance "Use these in moderation" (PCRM, 1997).

The first edition of the *Dietary Guidelines for Americans* was published in 1980 (USDA/HHS, 1980). To assist people in putting the Guidelines into practice, USDA released the Food Guide Pyramid (USDA, 1992).

The assumptions underlying the Food Guide Pyramid were that it would (1) promote overall health rather than treatment or prevention of a specific disease; (2) be based on up-to-date research on nutrient composition, foods commonly consumed, and nutrient recommendations such as the Recommended Dietary Allowances (RDAs) and the Dietary Reference Intakes (DRIs); (3) address the

171

total diet; (4) be useful to the target audience—the consumer; (5) be realistic; (6) be flexible; (7) be practical; and (8) be evolutionary.

The Food Guide Pyramid is based on the 1989 RDAs (NRC, 1989) and the 1990 Dietary Guidelines (Welsh et al., 1993) and incorporates data on foods used by the target population and data on nutrient composition of foods. The nutritional goals for the Pyramid are to provide a guide for individuals that is adequate in protein, vitamins, minerals, and dietary fiber, without excessive amounts of calories, fat, saturated fat, cholesterol, sodium, sugars, and alcohol (Shaw et al., 1996). It has been widely used as a resource for nutrition educators. As science advances, the Pyramid, as with other dietary guidance programs, should be reassessed to see that it meets current nutrition recommendations.

Canada's Food Guide to Healthy Eating

Canada's Food Guide to Healthy Eating (Health Canada, 1991) was developed from the Nutrition Recommendations (Health Canada, 1990b) and Canada's Guidelines for Healthy Eating (Health Canada, 1990a), through the work of technical groups and task forces, consumer research, and consultations with stakeholder groups. It provides details on daily food selection to meet nutritional needs of individuals aged 4 years and over and is designed for the general public with a reading level of grade seven.

The Food Guide is presented as a tear sheet with a consumer-oriented booklet, *Using the Food Guide* (Health Canada, 1997), which explains the concepts of the tear sheet. Nutrition professionals engaged in health promotion have also developed fact sheets to assist in using the Food Guide.

Nutritionists working with specific cultural groups or those with special dietary preferences, including Indigenous Peoples, have developed food guides that incorporate the local, cultural foods. An example is the *Food Guide for the Northwest Territories* (Northwest Territories Aboriginal Head Start Program, 2002). The Canadian guides are also updated as new science and better understanding of nutritional needs become available.

Uses of Food Guides in Planning for Individuals

The U.S. Food Guide Pyramid contains basic information needed for an individual to plan a day's food choices. It lists major food groups and subgroups, the ranges in numbers of servings suggested, and the amounts to count as a serving for each group. It also gives a range of servings intended to meet various caloric needs.

Canada's Food Guide to Healthy Eating can be used for different people in various life stages by attention to the top statement and the side bar describing number of servings (a lower and higher number of servings are given). Practitioners counseling individuals or individuals themselves can adjust the recommendation for age, body size, gender, activity level, pregnancy, breast-feeding, and individual variation. The Canadian Food Guide assumes that choosing foods according to the Guide can provide all nutrients needed for good health of most people. It recommends that supplements for special needs (e.g., for iron and folate during pregnancy) should be chosen after consultation with a physician or dietitian (Health Canada, 1997).

A physiological counterpart to *Canada's Food Guide to Healthy Eating* is the *Handbook for Canada's Physical Activity Guide to Healthy Active Living* (Health Canada, 1998). This guide provides a simple, consistent set of guidelines to achieve health benefits by being physically active. Silhouette figures on the Food Guide refer to the Vitality program, which integrates guidance (enjoy eating well, being active, and feeling good about oneself) that leads to an enhanced quality of life and maintenance of healthy weight.

FOOD LABELING AND NUTRIENT CONTENT CLAIMS

Food labels are an important and direct means of communicating product information between buyers (including the consumer) and sellers. They provide basic product information (e.g., name, ingredients, grade, etc.); they may provide health, safety, and nutrition information; and they serve as a vehicle for food marketing, promotion, and competition such as nutrition claims.

Development of Nutrition Labels—United States

In 1969 the White House Conference on Food, Nutrition, and Health recommended that the federal government consider developing a system for identifying the nutritional qualities of food. In 1973 the Food and Drug Administration (FDA) issued regulations requiring nutrition labeling on foods that contained one or more added nutrients or that had a label or advertising that included claims about the food's nutritional properties or its usefulness in the daily diet. The term "U.S. RDA" was also established at that time by FDA as the food label reference values for vitamins, minerals, and protein to be used in the companion voluntary nutrition labeling program resulting from this legislation. The U.S. RDAs were based on the adult age and gender groups with the highest values in the 1968 Recommended Dietary Allowances established for various population groups (NRC, 1968). Nutrition labeling took effect in 1975 for foods containing added nutrients or advertising claims and became voluntary for almost all other foods.

In 1990, Congress passed the Nutrition Labeling and Education Act, which required nutrition labeling for most foods (except meat and poultry) and authorized the use of nutrient content claims and appropriate FDA-approved health claims. These rules went into effect in 1994. In addition, voluntary nutrition information programs became effective in 1992. Nutrition information was made available under FDA's voluntary point-of-purchase nutrition information program for many raw foods, including the 20 most frequently eaten raw fruits, vegetables, and fish, and under USDA's program for the 45 best-selling cuts of meat.

Figure B-1 presents the Nutrition Facts panel that appears on current labels in the United States. The label reference value, Daily Value (DV), comprises two sets of dietary standards: the Daily Reference Values (DRVs) and Reference Daily Intakes (RDIs). Only the Daily Value term appears on the label. DRVs have been established for macronutrients that are sources of energy: fat, saturated fat, total carbohydrate (including fiber), and protein, as well as for cholesterol, sodium, and potassium.

DRVs for the energy-producing nutrients are based on an intake of 2,000 calories per day. This level was chosen, in part, because it approximates the caloric requirements for postmenopausal women, the life stage and gender group that has the highest risk for excessive intake of calories and fat.

DRVs for the energy-producing nutrients and fiber are calculated as follows:

- fat based on 30 percent of calories
- saturated fat based on 10 percent of calories
- carbohydrate based on 60 percent of calories
- protein based on 10 percent of calories (the DRV for protein applies only to adults and children over 4 years of age; RDIs for protein for special groups have been established)
- fiber based on 11.5 g of fiber per 1,000 calories

The DRVs for some nutrients represent the uppermost limit that is considered desirable under current public health recommendations. For example, the DRVs for total fat, saturated fat, cholesterol,

Nutrition Facts

Serving Size 1 cup (228g)
Serving Per Container 2

Amount Per Serving

Calories 250   Calories from Fat 110

	% Daily Value*
Total Fat 12g	18%
Saturated Fat 3g	15%
Cholesterol 30mg	10%
Sodium 470mg	20%
Total Carbohydrate 31g	10%
Dietary Fiber 0g	0%
Sugars 5g	
Protein 5g	

Vitamin A	4%
Vitamin C	2%
Calcium	20%
Iron	4%

* Percent Daily Values are based on a 2,000 calorie diet. Your Daily Values may be higher or lower depending on your calorie needs:

	Calories:	2,000	2,500
Total Fat	Less than	65g	80g
Sat Fat	Less than	20g	25g
Cholesterol	Less than	300mg	300mg
Sodium	Less than	2,400mg	2,400mg
Total Carbohydrate		300g	375g
Dietary Fiber		25g	30g

FIGURE B-1 U.S. food label.
SOURCE: FDA (2000).

and sodium are less than 65 g, 20 g, 300 mg, and 2,400 mg, respectively.

Daily Values—Reference Daily Intakes

The percent of DV stated on food labels for vitamins and minerals is based on the RDIs. The term RDI replaces the term U.S. RDA in current food labeling. However, most of the RDI values are the same as the U.S. RDAs that were provided on food labels in the past, and thus are also based on the 1968 RDAs. RDI values have also been established for nutrients for which RDAs were not established in 1968 (e.g., vitamin K, chromium). The RDI term was adopted to avoid confusion that might arise between the U.S. RDA used on food labels and the RDAs published by the National Academy of Sciences.

On the current label's "Nutrition Facts" panel, manufacturers are required to provide information on certain nutrients. The mandatory (underlined) and voluntary components and the order in which they must appear are listed in Box B-1.

The nutrients that are required on the label were selected because they address today's health concerns. The order in which they must appear was designed to reflect the priority of the then current dietary recommendations.

The nutrition information is presented in a defined serving size, which is the amount of food customarily eaten at one time. The serving sizes that appear on food labels are based on lists of Reference Amounts Customarily Consumed Per Eating Occasion, established by FDA (1999).

Current Nutrient Content Claims—United States

The following is a list of core terms that may be used to describe the level of a nutrient in a food under current regulations (FDA, 1999).

- *Free.* This term means that a product contains no amount of, or only trivial or "physiologically inconsequential" amounts of, one or more of these components: fat, saturated fat, cholesterol, sodium, sugars, and calories.
- *Low.* This term can be used on foods that can be eaten frequently without exceeding dietary guidelines for one or more of these components: fat, saturated fat, cholesterol, sodium, and calories. Thus, descriptors are low fat: 3 g or less per serving; low saturated fat: 1 g or less per serving; low sodium: 140 mg or less per serving; very low sodium: 35 mg or less per serving; low cholesterol: 20 mg or less and 2 g or less of saturated fat per serving; low calorie: 40 calories or less per serving.
- *Lean and extra lean.* These terms can be used to describe the fat content of meat, poultry, seafood, and game meats. Lean: less than 10 g of fat, 4.5 g or less of saturated fat, and less than 95 mg of cholesterol per serving and per 100 g; extra lean: less than 5 g of fat, less than 2 g of saturated fat, and less than 95 mg of cholesterol per serving and per 100 g.

BOX B-1 Nutrients on the U.S. Nutrition Facts Panel

- <u>total calories</u>
- <u>calories from fat</u>
- calories from saturated fat
- <u>total fat</u>
- <u>saturated fat</u>
- polyunsaturated fat
- monounsaturated fat
- <u>cholesterol</u>
- <u>sodium</u>
- potassium
- <u>total carbohydrate</u>
- <u>dietary fiber</u>
- soluble fiber
- insoluble fiber
- <u>sugars</u>

- sugar alcohol (for example, the sugar substitutes xylitol, mannitol, and sorbitol)
- other carbohydrate (the difference between total carbohydrate and the sum of dietary fiber and sugars)
- <u>protein</u>
- <u>vitamin A</u>
- percent of vitamin A present as β-carotene
- <u>vitamin C</u>
- <u>calcium</u>
- <u>iron</u>
- other essential vitamins and minerals

NOTE: Underlined components are required to appear on the panel.
SOURCE: FDA (1999).

- *High.* This term can be used if the food contains 20 percent or more of the DV for a particular nutrient in one serving.
- *Good source.* This term means that one serving of a food contains 10 to 19 percent of the DV for a particular nutrient.
- *Reduced.* This term means that a nutritionally altered product contains at least 25 percent less of a nutrient or calories than the regular, or reference, product. However, a "reduced" claim cannot be made on a product if its reference food already meets the requirement for a "low" claim.
- *Less.* This term means that a food, whether altered or not, contains 25 percent less of a nutrient or calories than the reference food.

Development of Food Labels—Canada

Since 1961 the Guide for Food Manufacturers and Advertisers has been the reference document on policies and regulations for the labeling and advertising of foods in Canada (CFIA, 1996). The current Guide to Food Labelling and Advertising (CFIA, 1996) provides labeling and advertising requirements, policies, and guide-lines that deal with statements and claims made for foods, including alcoholic beverages. Guidelines and provisions set out in the Food and Drugs Act and Food and Drugs Regulations, the Consumer Packaging and Labeling Act (CPLA), and other relevant legislation are provided. The responsibility for the administration of food-related provisions in the CPLA was transferred to the Canadian Food Inspection Agency in 1999.

Nutrition labeling in Canada has been voluntary, but under new regulations it has become mandatory on prepacked foods, with few exceptions. The nutrition label has a consistent format and always includes information on calories and the following 13 nutrients: fat, saturated fat, trans fat, cholesterol, sodium, carbohydrate, fiber, sugars, protein, vitamin A, vitamin C, calcium, and iron. Nutrient content is declared for a stated serving size, which may be different than that noted on the food guide. Vitamins and minerals are expressed as percent of a DV. Initially, DVs will be the same as the Recommended Daily Intakes that were developed for food labeling only, and are based on the highest Recommended Nutrient Intakes (RNIs) for individuals aged 2 and above from the 1983 Canadian RNIs, excluding needs during pregnancy and lactation. Figure B-2 provides an example of the new label, which is similar to the U.S. Nutrition Facts label.

Current Nutrient Content Claims—Canada

Amendments to the Canadian Food and Drugs Regulations (CFIA, 1996) regulate the compositional criteria and specific labeling requirements for all permitted nutrient content claims. Permitted nutrient content claims include claims that a product is "free" of a substance (e.g., fat-free, free of trans fatty acids, calorie-free, sugar-free); is "low in" or "reduced or lower in" a substance (e.g., calories, fat, saturated fatty acids, trans fatty acids, cholesterol, sugar); has "no added" sodium, salt, or sugar, or is a "source of," a "high source of," a "very high source of," or an "excellent source of" a nutrient (e.g., protein, fiber, vitamins, and minerals). In each case, composi-tional criteria must be met. For example, a food claiming it is "cho-lesterol-free" would have less than 2 mg of cholesterol per standard serving size, and would also need to meet the criteria to be "low in saturated fatty acids."

The proposed amendments to the Food and Drugs Regulations will also allow for five diet-related health claims to be made relative to reduced risk of high blood pressure, osteoporosis, heart disease,

Nutrition Facts

Per 1 cup (264g)

Amount	% Daily Value
Calories 260	
Fat 13g	20%
Saturated Fat 3g + Trans Fat 2g	25%
Cholesterol 30mg	
Sodium 660mg	28%
Carbohydrate 31g	10%
Fibre 0g	0%
Sugars 5g	
Protein 5g	
Vitamin A 4% ▪ Vitamin C 2%	
Calcium 15% ▪ Iron 4%	

FIGURE B-2 Canadian food label.
SOURCE: Health Canada (2002).

some types of cancer, and dental caries. The amendments specify the wording for the permitted health claim and the compositional criteria that foods would have to meet in order to qualify for the claim.

DIETARY GUIDELINES IN THE UNITED STATES AND CANADA

The current U.S. and Canadian dietary guidelines are not generally related to micronutrients, with the exception of guidelines pertaining to "variety." The intent of these guidelines (i.e., Canadian "Enjoy a variety of foods" and U.S. "Let the Pyramid guide your food choices") is to promote a greater likelihood of meeting recommended intakes of all nutrients through choosing a variety of foods.

Dietary Guidelines for Americans

The fifth edition of the *Dietary Guidelines for Americans* was released in 2000 (USDA/HHS, 2000). The focus of the Guidelines is on good health, including reducing risk for chronic diseases. The Guidelines are based on fitness, the Food Pyramid, food safety, and the ability to choose foods sensibly.

The concept of the Guidelines began with the 1977 Dietary Goals of the United States developed by the Senate Select Committee on Nutrition and Human Needs. These goals focused on reducing the incidence of chronic disease rather than on reducing nutritional deficiencies, and recommended quantifiable targets for carbohydrates, fats, and cholesterol in the American diet.

The *Dietary Guidelines for Americans* (Box B-2), developed jointly by USDA and the Department of Health and Human Services (HHS), was first published in 1980 and subsequently revised in 1985, 1990, 1995, and 2000. It provides recommendations based on current scientific knowledge about the association between dietary intake and risk of major chronic diseases. The National Nutrition Monitoring and Related Research Act of 1990 (Public Law 101-445, Title III) required publication of the Guidelines at least every five years beginning in 1985. This legislation also required review by the secretaries of USDA and HHS of all federal dietary guidance-related publications for the general public.

The Guidelines serve as a framework for consumer education messages. They also form the basis of federal food, nutrition educa-

---

BOX B-2 Dietary Guidelines for Americans

Aim for a healthy weight.
Be physically active each day.
Let the Pyramid guide your food choices.
Eat a variety of grains daily, especially whole grains.
Choose a variety of fruits and vegetables daily.
Keep food safe to eat.
Choose a diet that is low in saturated fat and cholesterol and moderate in total fat.
Choose beverages and foods to moderate your intake of sugars.
Choose and prepare foods with less salt.
If you drink alcoholic beverages, do so in moderation.

SOURCE: USDA/HHS (2000).

tion, and information programs and are used for individual counseling, in group education settings such as schools and outpatient settings, and for general food and nutrition planning. The Guidelines are widely available through professional nutritionists' and dietitians' associations, health clinics, government-sponsored health settings, the food industry, and the media.

Nutrition Recommendations for Canadians

In Canada, national guidelines for consideration of nutrition programs and policies have been in effect for more than 60 years. They have been used by professional and other organizations, government at all levels, the food and food service industry, and by individual consumers. The most recent review of Canada's national nutrition guidelines took place from 1987 to 1989 by two committees: one that considered revisions to the RNIs and one that considered consumer advice and implementation strategies. This work resulted in the current Nutrition Recommendations (Health Canada, 1990b), and, ultimately, *Canada's Food Guide to Healthy Eating* (Health Canada, 1991). The Nutrition Recommendations (Box B-3)

BOX B-3 Canadian Nutrition Recommendations

- The Canadian diet should provide energy consistent with the maintenance of body weight within the recommended range.
- The Canadian diet should include essential nutrients in amounts recommended.
- The Canadian diet should include no more than 30% of energy as fat (33 g/1,000 kcal or 39 g/5,000 kJ) and no more than 10% as saturated fat (11 g/1,000 kcal or 13 g/5,000 kJ).
- The Canadian diet should provide 55% of energy as carbohydrate (138 g/ 1,000 kcal or 165 g/5,000 kJ) from a variety of sources.
- The sodium content of the Canadian diet should be reduced.
- The Canadian diet should include no more than 5% of total energy as alcohol, or two drinks daily, whichever is less.
- The Canadian diet should contain no more caffeine than the equivalent of four regular cups of coffee per day.
- Community water supplies containing less that 1 mg/L should be fluoridated to that level.

SOURCE: Health Canada (1990b).

BOX B-4 Canada's Guidelines for Healthy Eating

- Enjoy a VARIETY of foods.
- Emphasize cereals, breads, other grain products, vegetables, and fruit.
- Choose lower-fat dairy products, leaner meats, and foods prepared with little or no fat.
- Achieve and maintain a healthy body weight by enjoying regular physical activity and healthy eating.
- Limit salt, alcohol, and caffeine.

SOURCE: Health Canada (1991).

---

were directed to health professionals and describe desirable characteristics of the diet in relatively technical terms. These recommendations were "translated" to Canada's Guidelines for Healthy Eating (Box B-4), which provide key messages directed to consumers. These guidelines were designed to be action-oriented, positive statements that would lead to the selection of diets that meet the Nutrition Recommendations.

C

The Target Nutrient Density
of a Single Food

As discussed in Chapter 4, planning for groups that include individuals with different nutrient requirements as well as different energy requirements is complicated. This is because individuals vary not only with respect to the amount of food they consume, but also in their choice of foods. However, if all individuals in the group consume a diet consisting of a single, nutritionally complete food (e.g., in an emergency feeding situation), then planners need to account only for the variability across individuals in the amount of food they consume. In this simplified scenario, the target nutrient density in a food can be directly obtained from the distribution of requirements expressed as a density, as described below.

The first step in determining intake of a diet composed of a single food (or of a mix of foods with similar nutrient density) is to obtain a target nutrient density of the food for each subgroup in the heterogeneous group.

Given a distribution of usual energy intakes in the subgroup, what is the target density of the nutrient in the food so that the prevalence of nutrient inadequacy in the subgroup is low? Calculation of the target nutrient density in a single (nutritionally complete) food to achieve a certain acceptable prevalence of inadequate intakes is simple if the distribution of density requirements is available. The concept of a distribution of requirements of a nutrient expressed as a density is now introduced, because it makes the planning of intakes of a diet consisting of a single food a relatively simple task even for a heterogeneous group.

THE DISTRIBUTION OF REQUIREMENTS FOR A NUTRIENT EXPRESSED AS A DENSITY

To obtain the distribution of requirements expressed as a nutrient density, it is necessary to know the distributions of nutrient requirements and the distributions of usual energy intakes in the various subgroups that comprise the target group. For most nutrients for which an Estimated Average Requirement (EAR) has been established, the distributions of requirements have been implicitly assumed to be normal, with mean (and median) equal to the EAR, and the coefficient of variation (CV) of 10 percent (except for niacin, copper, and molybdenum, which have a CV of 15 percent, and vitamin A and iodine, which have a CV of 20 percent [IOM 1997, 1998a, 2000b, 2001]). Even if a nutrient has a skewed requirement distribution, as in the case of iron and protein, the method introduced in this section can still be applied. Following the discussion presented in Chapter 4, it is assumed that estimates of the distributions of usual energy intakes are available for each of the subgroups that comprise the heterogeneous group of interest.

The approach described below to derive the distribution of requirements of a nutrient expressed as a density is flexible. It can be used for any nutrient (including iron, for which the requirement distribution is known to be nonnormal). Because reliable information to derive the distribution of nutrient density requirements when nutrient requirements and energy intakes are not independent is not available, this approach assumes independence.

To derive the requirement distribution of a nutrient expressed as a density, proceed as follows:

1. Simulate a large number n of requirements from the distribution of nutrient requirements in the group. For most nutrients, this implies drawing n random values from a normal distribution with a mean equal to the EAR of the nutrient in the subgroup and a CV equal to 10 percent of the EAR (15 or 20 percent for some nutrients).

2. Simulate a large number n of usual energy intakes from the distribution of usual energy intakes in the subgroup, or in a group that is believed to be reasonably similar in energy intakes to the subgroup of interest.

3. For each pair of simulated nutrient requirements and usual energy intakes, construct the ratio *nutrient requirement/usual energy intake*. The distribution of these n ratios is an estimate of the requirement distribution of the nutrient expressed as a density.

As an example, the distribution of vitamin C requirements for nonsmoking women aged 19 to 50 years is assumed to be normal with an EAR of 60 mg/day (IOM, 2000b) and a standard deviation of 10 percent of the EAR, or 6 mg/day. For boys aged 14 to 18 years, the distribution of vitamin C requirements is normal with an EAR of 63 mg/day and standard deviation of 6.3 mg/day. For energy, this example uses normal distributions with means equal to 1,900 kcal/day and 2,300 kcal/day for women and boys, respectively, and a CV of 20 percent to represent the distributions of usual energy intakes in each of the two subgroups. (In practice, the actual usual energy intake distributions would be used to construct the distribution of nutrient requirements expressed as densities. However, the mean energy intakes and CV of energy intake used in this example closely correspond to those that would be obtained from an analysis of the 1994–1996 Continuing Survey of Food Intakes by Individuals [ARS, 1998].)

The Statistical Analysis System program used to derive the distribution of vitamin C requirements expressed as a density in each of the two subgroups is given at the end of this appendix. A sample size of $n = 10,000$ values of vitamin C requirements and of usual energy intakes for each of the two groups was simulated and the ratio was constructed as described in step 3 above. The resulting two density requirement distributions are shown in Figure C-1.

Notice that the two density requirement distributions shown in the figure are skewed, even though the distributions of vitamin C requirements and of usual energy intakes were assumed to be normal. Notice too that it is possible to compute the mean, median, or any percentile of the derived requirement distributions for the nutrient densities because through the simulation, there are many observations (in this example, 10,000) from each of the distributions.

THE PERCENTILE METHOD TO DERIVE THE TARGET NUTRIENT DENSITY OF A SINGLE FOOD

The target nutrient density of a single food can be directly established from the distribution of nutrient requirements expressed as density that was derived in the preceding section.

In the following illustrations, 3 percent is used as the desired prevalence of inadequate intake. Continuing with the example used earlier, consider the problem of estimating the target vitamin C density in a single food so that the prevalence of inadequate vitamin C intakes in nonsmoking women aged 19 to 50 years and boys

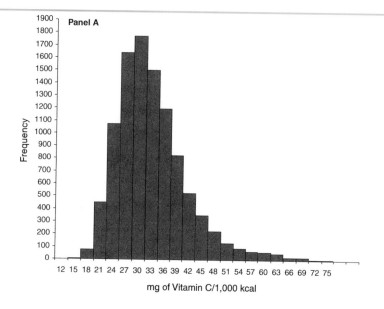

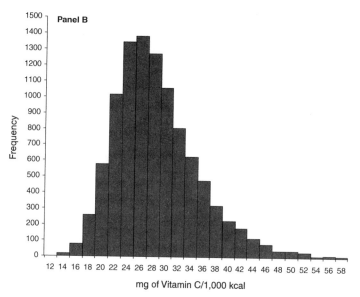

FIGURE C-1 Simulated requirement distributions of vitamin C expressed as densities for nonsmoking women aged 19 to 50 years (Panel A) and for boys aged 14 to 18 years (Panel B). The distributions were constructed using the SAS program presented at the end of this appendix and using information on requirements of vitamin C for the two subgroups (IOM, 2000b). The usual energy intake distributions used in the example are hypothetical.

aged 14 to 18 years does not exceed 3 percent. To obtain the appropriate density, it is necessary to estimate the 97th percentiles of each of the density distributions so only 3 percent would have requirements above this density. In this example, the values obtained are 63.6 mg/1,000 kcal and 42.9 mg/1,000 kcal for women and boys, respectively (see Figure C-1). That is, to ensure that the prevalence of inadequate vitamin C intakes among nonsmoking women aged 19 to 50 years does not exceed 3 percent, the planner must provide a food with a vitamin C density equal to 63.6 mg/1,000 kcal. In the case of boys aged 14 to 18 years, the target vitamin C density in the food is 42.9 mg/1,000 kcal.

To plan intakes of a single food in a heterogeneous group consisting of these two subgroups, the planner would provide a food with vitamin C of density at least 63.6 mg/1,000 kcal, the higher of the two target densities computed above. This is called the reference nutrient density, and is a key tool for planning diets for heterogeneous groups.

The reference nutrient density is defined as the highest target nutrient density among the subgroups in the group being planned for. It is designed to lead to an acceptable prevalence of nutrient inadequacy in the subgroup with the highest target nutrient density. For the entire group, the prevalence of inadequacy would be even lower.

By basing planning on the highest target nutrient density, the planner guarantees that the group with the highest density requirements will have its needs met. In the group with the lowest density requirements, in this case boys 14 to18 years of age, the prevalence of inadequate nutrient intakes will very likely be lower than the target. In fact, the target nutrient density of 63.6 mg of vitamin C/ 1,000 kcal is approximately equal to the 99.5 percentile of the density requirement distribution computed for the boys. Therefore, if the food provided has a vitamin C density of 63.6 mg/1,000 kcal, only about 0.5 percent of the boys in the group will have inadequate vitamin C intakes. This target nutrient density would also need to be evaluated to ensure an acceptably low prevalence of intakes above the Tolerable Upper Intake Level (UL) in the boys. The actual densities derived in this example are for illustration purposes only. In practice, the planner would use a better estimate of the distribution of energy intakes in the subgroups of interest.

The percentile method to obtain the reference nutrient density is very general in that there are essentially no underlying assumptions that must hold for the method to work well. In fact, in principle this approach does not even require that nutrient requirements and usual energy intakes be independent; however, in practice, the independence assumption is made as there is no reliable information that would allow statistical estimation of the joint distribution of nutrient requirement and usual energy intake. Because the derivation of the density requirement distribution and its desirable percentile is done by simulation, it is not even necessary to assume that the distribution of nutrient requirements or of usual energy intakes is normal. Therefore, this approach can be used for iron even though the distribution of requirements is known to be skewed (IOM, 2001).

This percentile approach applies only to planning scenarios where the target group consumes a single food item or mix of foods with very similar nutrient densities. In these scenarios, the variability in intakes across individuals in the heterogeneous group is due only to variability in the amounts of the food (or mix of foods) consumed. In most planning situations, however, individuals vary both in the amount of food consumed and in the choice of the foods they consume. If they choose from a selection of foods with different nutrient densities, then even if the average nutrient density is set as above, it is possible that some individuals will consume the lower-density food items, while others may consume the higher-density food items. When there is heterogeneity in food choices among individuals in a group, one cannot use this simple percentile approach to estimate the necessary food density that will guarantee a low risk of inadequacy for almost all individuals in the group.

MATHEMATICAL PROOF

A simple mathematical proof for the result is presented here. The symbol α is used to denote the nutrient density, or units of the nutrient per 1,000 kcal.

The percentile method attempts to provide an answer to the following question: Given a certain distribution of usual energy intakes, what is the target density, α, of the nutrient so that the prevalence of nutrient inadequacy in the group is low, for example, 2.5 percent?

The result proved below establishes that if the target prevalence of inadequacy is set at $p\%$, then α is the $(1 - p)$th percentile (the upper $[1 - p]$th point) of the distribution of the random variable *nutrient requirement/usual energy intake*.

Proof of Result

To prove that the result presented above is correct, some notation is introduced:

- The symbol x denotes requirement of the nutrient, and is a random variable with some known distribution.
- The symbol y denotes the usual energy intake in the group, and is also a random variable with some distribution.
- The symbol α is the target density or concentration of the nutrient in 1,000 kcal of the food under consideration. Given a usual energy intake equal to y, the target usual intake of the nutrient is equal to αy.

An individual does not have an adequate target intake of the nutrient if $\alpha y < x$, that is, if his or her target usual nutrient intake is less than his or her requirement.

Suppose one wanted to plan a nutrient density so that $p\%$ of the group consumes an adequate amount of the nutrient, given a certain distribution of energy intakes in the group.

Find $\alpha \in (0,1)$ such that

$$\Pr(\alpha y > x) = p \qquad (1)$$

If x is deleted from both sides of the inequality then equation (1) implies

$$\Pr(\alpha y - x > 0) = p$$

and, therefore

$$\Pr(\alpha - x/y > 0) = p$$

Then

$$\Pr(x/y < \alpha) = 1 - p \qquad (2)$$

But expression (2) says that α is larger than x/y with probability $1 - p$ and therefore α has to be the $(1 - p)$th percentile of the distribution of the ratio x/y (by definition of percentile).

Assumptions

The result is true for just about any case. The proof above requires only that x and y be positive. There are no conditions on the distributions of requirements and usual intakes; neither normality nor symmetry of the two distributions is required for the result to hold. In fact, it is not even necessary to assume that intakes and requirements are independent.

However, in order to obtain a numerical value for α, specific distributions for requirements of the nutrient and for energy intakes need to be chosen. Note that the result above holds even if the distribution of requirements happens to be skewed. Thus, the percentile method works for iron in menstruating women.

In the special case in which both the nutrient requirement and the energy intake distributions are normal, it is possible to derive an analytical expression for α.

SAS PROGRAM TO COMPUTE THE REQUIREMENT DISTRIBUTIONS EXPRESSED AS DENSITIES

The program below was used to obtain the two density requirement distributions shown in Figure C-1. Comments are given between /* and */ symbols. The integer numbers given in parentheses after the *rannor* statements are seeds to initialize the random number generators. Any value between 1 and 99999 can be used as a seed. The requirement distribution of a nutrient expressed as a density is needed to plan intakes of a single food or of a diet composed of various foods with similar nutrient density.

```
data one ;
do i = 1 to 10000 ; /* Start simulation of 10,000 vit C requirements
    and energy intakes */
vcreq_w = rannor(675)*6 + 60 ; /* women: vit C req ~ N(60, 6²) */
vcreq_b = rannor(903)*6.3 + 63 ; /*boys: vit C req ~ N(63, 6.3²) */
ereq_w = rannor(432)*380 + 1900 ; /* women: energy intake ~
    N(1900, 380²) */
ereq_b = rannor(500)*460 + 2300 ; /* boys: energy intake ~ N(2300,
    460²) */
ratio_w = (vcreq_w/ ereq_w)*1000 ; /* women: vit C requirements /
    1000 kcal */
ratio_b = (vcreq_b/ ereq_b)*1000 ; /* boys: vit C requirements /
    1000 kcal */
```

```
output ;
end ;
run ;

proc gchart data = one ; /* Obtain the charts in Figure C-1 */
vbar ratio_w ratio_b/ levels = 50 space = 0 ;
run ;

proc sort data = one ; by ratio_w ; /* women: obtain target density
     for single food */
run ;

data temp ; set one ; if _n_ = 9700 ; /* women: 97th percentile of density
     requirements */
run ;

proc print data = temp ; run ; /* women: print target density for
     single food */

proc sort data = one ; by ratio_b ; /* boys: obtain target density for
     single food */
run ;

data temp ; set one ; if _n_ = 9700 ; /* boys: 97th percentile of density
     requirements */
run ;

proc print data = temp ; run ; /* boys: print target density for single
     food */
```

D
Voluntary Nutrient Fortification

Fortification of foods with one or more micronutrients is used as a public health intervention intended to meet a defined population health problem. Perhaps the most widely cited example of successful fortification is the iodination of salt for the control and prevention of goiter and other iodine deficiency diseases (IDD). Salt iodination is now practiced in at least 107 countries, with an estimated overall coverage of 68 percent of households in those countries (ACC/SCN, 2000). Although IDD prevalence is falling rapidly, there are 130 countries in which IDD is still considered a public health problem. In Canada, fortification of free-running table salt is mandatory; in the United States, subject to state laws, it is voluntary. The iodination of salt continues to be actively promoted and has proven to be an extremely effective intervention in the iodine-deficient area of the Great Lakes basin of both countries. In the United States, the addition of niacin to cornmeal and flour for the control of pellagra, at one time endemic in the southeast, and the fluoridation of water to reduce dental caries have been clear success stories.

Efforts are now underway to achieve an equivalent success story for vitamin A and iron in developing countries. Technology for fortification is available but, because of the very limited use of processed foods, there is very limited opportunity for fortification in many of the countries most in need of fortified foods (IOM, 1998b).

In North America, a very large proportion of the food supply is processed, thus providing ample opportunity for fortification. The technology of fortification and preparation of nutrient premixes that are stable and do not cause taste, odor, or color changes are now available for a wide variety of products. The food industry thus can greatly increase the scope of fortification (more nutrients and more foods). However, with these advances in technology and greatly increased scope of opportunity comes the risk of overfortification.

In the past, when a clear public health problem was identified and only one or two foods were being fortified, the planning and monitoring of fortification was conceptually relatively easy. One could proceed along the lines exemplified for the mock fortification of fluid milk with vitamin A presented in Chapter 5. In the planning stage the potential benefit of nutrient addition, as well as the potential risk of excessive intake, could be predicted at a theoretical level. This could be done not only for the target groups where the public health problem was most severe, but also for other population segments likely to consume the fortified food. This is the type of preliminary planning that was done in the United States prior to increasing levels of fortification of bread flour with folate in the late 1990s. A defined public health problem existed, and only a few foods were targeted for the increased fortification.

Fortification planning has become complicated by three factors. First, as noted previously, the opportunity for fortification has increased tremendously and the number of foods involved has increased in the United States as manufacturers have implemented their own fortification decisions. Therefore, individuals may consume multiple sources of the fortificant. Second, the food industry is technologically ready to meet perceived needs for nutrients, and with nutrients for which the new recommended intakes may suggest increased need (IOM, 1997, 1998a, 2000b, 2001, 2002a), industry is anxious to respond. Third, there is an increased consumer awareness of nutrient composition of individual foods through nutrition labeling and a general rise in interest in nutrition and its potential health benefits. Over time, this has meant that labeled nutrient content and associated claims or inferred benefits have become important market influences. This places competitive pressure on the food industry to add more and larger amounts of nutrients to foods. Accordingly, the focus of nutrient fortification has shifted from carefully orchestrated and closely monitored interventions to address specified public health problems to a much less controlled and broader, non-orchestrated program of nutrient additions to meet market demands and competitive pressures. Where only a few fortified foods were marketed a few decades ago, there are now fortified and fabricated foods numbering in the thousands.

As an example, a recent study of U.S. food consumption (Berner et al., 2001) evaluated the impact of 246 different fortified foods on nutrient intakes of populations. Children were found to be the most likely to consume fortified foods with 70 to 80 percent of children aged 1 to 10 years consuming foods fortified with vitamins A and C, thiamin, folate, or iron. In contrast, only 34 to 38 percent of adult women consumed these foods. A similar situation in Germany was reported (Sichert-Helert et al., 1999) where children aged 2 to 14 years consumed 479 different fortified food products.

In both the United States and Canada, food fortification has created difficult problems for government agencies involved in public health monitoring. Canada is currently formulating a new policy on fortification and designing new regulations under that policy (Health Canada, 1999). The fundamental difficulty is that fortification regulations (minimum and maximum levels to be added, compulsory versus voluntary addition, etc.) relate to single foods or classes of commodities that are used interchangeably. For example, stimulated by concerns over vitamin D deficiencies and possible links between excessive vitamin D intake and cases of idiopathic hypercalcemia, Canadian regulations were modified to allow the addition of vitamin D to all types of milks, but to prohibit its addition to most other types of foods. The milk products were considered to be interchangeable and mutually exclusive.

The regulatory framework was developed to address the control of rickets in Canada, while at the same time avoiding the problem of infantile hypercalcemia, which had been attributed to excessive intakes of vitamin D (perhaps combined with high calcium intakes). This approach appeared to be effective in addressing the public health problem, but did not guarantee that every individual would ingest the recommended amount of vitamin D.

Many have urged that the regulations be eased to allow addition of vitamin D to a much wider range of foods, as is allowed in the United States. Such a relaxation of control would increase the likelihood that those who drank very little or no milk could get adequate vitamin D from another food. However, there is also the concern that excessive intakes may result if individuals consume several fortified foods. Thus, a dilemma exists for regulatory agencies.

As stated earlier, with compulsory fortification of only a few foods, mock fortification studies (such as the vitamin A example in Chapter 5) can be conducted to assess expected benefits and potential risks associated with different levels of fortification. However, because the number of fortified foods has increased, it is no longer possible to run meaningful mock fortification scenarios.

Furthermore, it has not been possible for food composition databases to stay current with the increasing numbers of foods fortified with an array of different nutrients added at different levels. Intake data collected in national surveys would have to carry brand names and perhaps manufacturing dates in order to have accurate assessments of intake for use in planning fortification programs. It is not currently possible to use large national dietary studies to monitor the public health impacts of fortification.

An additional concern was highlighted by Whittaker and colleagues (2001) who examined iron and folate levels in 29 fortified breakfast cereals. The analyzed content of iron in these cereals ranged from 80 to 190 percent of label values, with 21 of the 29 cereals containing 120 percent or more above label values. Analyzed values for folate ranged from 98 to 320 percent of label values. In addition, label values were based on a serving size of 30 g, but the median measured serving size was 47 g for women and 61 g for men. Consequently, intakes of iron and folate would be considerably higher than what would be estimated based on standard portion sizes and nutrition label information, with the prevalence of intakes greater than the Tolerable Upper Intake Level being much higher than predicted.

Food fortification thus has become a risk–risk situation that requires balancing concerns of inadequate intakes with concerns of excessive intakes. One approach to solve this problem is to tightly regulate additional fortification efforts, but then the individuals who do not consume the existing fortified products would not have other sources available to achieve adequate dietary intake. Another option is to allow industry to respond to market demand and increase fortification, but then the risk of excessive levels of intake among those consuming multiple fortified products or high amounts of single fortified foods increases.

Nutritionists generally do not think in terms of adequacy of individual foods. Rather, limits of intake (inadequacy to excess) are based on "habitual dietary intakes," or the self-selected mix of foods consumed over long periods by individuals. Fortification regulations have to relate to single foods or groups of foods. The increasing use of over-the-counter pharmaceutical supplements and dietary supplements, potentially by the same health-conscious people who scan nutrition labels for foods with the highest available nutrient levels, must also be factored into decisions on nutrient fortification policy.

E

Adjustment of Observed Intake Data to Estimate the Distribution of Usual Intakes in a Group

An individual's actual intake varies considerably from one day to the next, but it is usual or long-term average intakes that are of interest in assessing and planning dietary intakes to ensure nutrient adequacy for individuals or groups. As explained in a previous report (IOM, 2000a), serious error in the assessment of nutrient inadequacy or excess can occur if the dietary intake data examined do not reflect usual intakes. This poses a major obstacle to the assessment of an individual's nutrient intake because his or her usual intake is generally poorly estimated from only a few days of observation, yet more extensive data collection is rarely feasible. Assessments of nutrient adequacy among groups are facilitated by the availability of statistical adjustment procedures to estimate the distribution of usual intakes from observed intakes, as long as more than one day of intake data has been collected for at least a representative subsample of the group. These procedures do not yield estimates of usual intake for particular individuals in the group, but the adjusted distribution of intakes is appropriate for use in analyses of the prevalence of inadequate or excess intakes in the group.

In recent years a number of different statistical procedures have been developed to estimate the distribution of usual intakes from repeated short-term measurements (Hoffmann et al., 2002). Two commonly used adjustment procedures are described here: the National Research Council (NRC) method and the Iowa State University (ISU) method. Both procedures are based on a common conceptual foundation, but the ISU method includes a number of statistical enhancements that make it more appropriate for use with large population surveys. The NRC method is simpler and may be more appropriate than the ISU method for use with small samples (those with less than 40 to 50 individuals). However, neither method is without limitations.

THE NATIONAL RESEARCH COUNCIL METHOD

Conceptual Underpinnings

In assessing nutrient adequacy it is necessary to estimate usual intake. However, usual intake cannot be inferred from measures of observed intake without error. For any one individual,

Observed intake = usual intake + measurement error

The observed variance ($V_{observed}$) of a distribution of intakes for a group based on one or more days of intake data per individual is the sum of the variance in true usual intakes of the individuals who comprise the group (e.g., the between-person or interindividual variance, $V_{between}$) and the error in the measurement of individuals' true usual intakes. Error arises both because of the normal variation in individuals' intakes from one day to the next and because of random error in the measurement of intake on any one day. It is referred to as the within-person, day-to-day, or intraindividual variance (V_{within}) (NRC, 1986).

$$V_{observed} = V_{between} + V_{within} + V_{underreporting}$$

The observed distribution of intakes will be wider and flatter than the true distribution of usual intakes as a result of the presence of within-person variance. However, assuming that the within-person variation is random in nature, the estimate of mean intake for the group will not be influenced by this variance.

If multiple days of intake data per individual are averaged, and the distribution of intakes in the group is constructed from the means of each individual's multiple intakes, then the error variance (e.g., within-person variance) diminishes as a function of the number of days of intake data per person. Thus, as the number of days of data per person increases, the distribution of observed intakes (expressed as the individuals' observed mean intakes over the days of data collection) becomes a better and better approximation of the true distribution of usual intakes in the group.

The NRC method (NRC, 1986) is typically applied to a data set comprising multiple days of intake data for a sample of individuals, ideally with an equal number of observations per individual. This method of estimating the distribution of usual intakes works by first partitioning the observed variance into its between- and within-person components, and then shifting each point in the observed distribution closer to the mean by a function of the ratio of the square roots of the between-person variance ($V_{between}$) and observed variance ($V_{observed}$). In this way, the method attempts to remove the effect of within-person variation on the observed distribution. The variance of the adjusted distribution should represent $V_{between}$.

Application

The steps in the NRC method are outlined below. The method is illustrated using data on the zinc intakes of 46 women recorded over three, nonconsecutive, 24-hour dietary intake recalls (a subsample of women drawn from a earlier study by Tarasuk and Beaton [1999]).

Step 1. Examine normality of distribution and transform data if necessary.

This adjustment procedure depends on the properties of a normal distribution, yet the observed distribution of intakes for most nutrients is likely to be positively skewed. This is because the distribution is naturally truncated at 0 (i.e., reported intakes cannot fall below this value) but has no limit at the upper end. Thus it is imperative that the normality of the 1-day intake data be assessed. (This can be accomplished through the NORMAL option in PROC UNIVARIATE in SAS.) If departures from normality are detected, the data should be transformed to approximate a normal distribution. The most appropriate transformation will depend on the shape of the original distribution; it may have a logarithm, square root, or cubed root relationship.

Note that for this example, the assessment of normality is conducted on all 138 days of recall data (e.g., 46 women multiplied by 3 days). The Shapiro-Wilk statistic, W, provides one measure of the normality of the data (Tarasuk and Beaton, 1999). For the raw data, $W = 0.85$ (versus a value of 1 for normally distributed data), and the distribution departs significantly from normality ($p < 0.0001$). A visual inspection of the plotted data reveals that they are right-skewed. Through a process of trial and error, a more normal distribution is achieved by applying a cubed root transformation to these data.

The W of the transformed data is 0.99 ($p = 0.1812$). The next two steps in this adjustment procedure are conducted using the transformed data.

Step 2. Estimate the within- and between-person variance.

Some statistical packages have procedures for partitioning the variance of the observed data into the within- and between-person variance components (e.g., PROC VARCOMP in SAS). This can also be easily accomplished using the analysis of variance procedures available in most statistical packages by conducting a simple one-way ANOVA with subject ID included as a categorical or class variable. A sample program for SAS is presented at the end of this appendix. When the raw data are transformed to better resemble a normal distribution, this step is conducted on the transformed data.

Two values are extracted from the ANOVA output. The mean square error or unexplained variance (e.g., the variance in the observed daily intakes that is not accounted for by between-subject differences) represents the within-subject variance in the 1-day data. The mean square model (e.g., the mean square associated with the subject ID variable entered into the ANOVA) represents the observed variance of the 1-day data. Because the adjustment procedure is applied to an individual subject's mean intakes over the period of observation, both the mean square model and mean square error need to be divided by the mean number of days of intake data per subject to obtain the $V_{observed}$ and V_{within} for this distribution (e.g., $V_{observed}$ = mean square model/n and V_{within} = mean square error/n). $V_{between}$ can be estimated by subtracting V_{within} from $V_{observed}$, as follows:

$$V_{between} = (\text{mean square model} - \text{mean square error})/n$$

where n is the mean number of days of intake data per subject in the sample. $V_{between}$ represents the "true" variance of the distribution of usual intakes. Each of these variance estimates can be expressed as a standard deviation by simply taking the square root of the variance.

Table E-1 presents the output for the ANOVA procedure as applied to this example. The mean number of days of intake data per subject is three. In this example, $V_{observed}$ = 0.24633584/3, V_{within} = 0.13375542/3 and $V_{between}$ = (0.24633584 − 0.13375542)/3.

TABLE E-1 ANOVA of Zinc Intake of 46 Adult Women, Shown for Data Transformed Using Cubed Roots

Source	Degrees of Freedom	Sum of Squares	Mean Square	F Value	Pr > F
Model	45	11.08511265	0.24633584	1.84	< 0.0069
Error	92	12.30549834	0.13375542		
Corrected total	137	23.39061099			

Step 3. Adjust individual subjects' mean intakes to estimate the distribution of usual intakes.

Each subject's mean intake is now adjusted by applying the following formula:

$$\text{Adjusted intake} = [(\text{subject's mean} - \text{group mean}) \times (SD_{between}/SD_{observed})] + \text{group mean}$$

where $SD_{between}$ is the square root of $V_{between}$ and $SD_{observed}$ is the square root of $V_{observed}$. This equation effectively moves each point in the distribution of observed intakes closer to the group mean, but it does not shift the group mean. If the distribution of 1-day data was transformed prior to partitioning the variance (Step 2), the equation is applied to the individual subject and group means calculated from the transformed data (Step 3), and the resultant distribution needs to be transformed back prior to use (see Step 4). If the data were not transformed, however, the adjusted intakes calculated from this equation now represent the estimated distribution of usual intakes.

Step 4. If the original data have been transformed, transform the adjusted intake back to the original units.

If the original data were transformed in order to satisfy the necessary assumption of normality, the adjusted data need to be transformed back into the original units prior to their use for nutrient assessment. Back-transforming refers to the application of the inverse function of the original transformation. In this example, the original data were transformed using cubed roots; the back transformation raises subject's adjusted intakes to the power of three. The process of transforming data, adjusting it, and then back-transforming it is

TABLE E-2 Observed Distribution of 3-day Mean Zinc Intakes (mg) and Estimated (Adjusted) Distribution of Usual Intakes for a Sample of 46 Women

Zinc Intake	Mean	Standard Deviation	25th Percentile	50th Percentile	75th Percentile
Observed 3-day means	8.84	3.58	6.11	8.49	10.97
Adjusted intake	8.03	2.20	6.58	8.15	9.33

necessary to preserve the shape of the original distribution for analysis purposes while removing the within-person variance.

Table E-2 presents a comparison of the distribution of the observed subjects' 3-day means to the adjusted intake. The variance of the adjusted intake distribution is substantially less than the variance of the distribution of the observed 3-day means, as evidenced by the adjusted intake's lower standard deviation. In addition, the distance between the 25th and 75th percentiles of the adjusted intake distribution is closer to its mean than that of the observed 3-day mean.

If the Estimated Average Requirement (EAR) cut-point method is applied to the adjusted distribution to assess the prevalence of inadequate zinc intakes among this sample, an estimated 26 percent of women (12/46) appear to have inadequate intakes (12 of the 46 adjusted means were below the EAR for zinc for women of 6.8 mg/day). This is lower than the 28 percent prevalence of inadequacy that would be estimated from the unadjusted data.

Special Considerations

Two features of the NRC method deserve special note because they pose challenges to analysts wanting to use this approach. First is the requirement for normally distributed data, and the second is the handling of incomplete data.

Normality

As noted earlier, the NRC method hinges on having normally distributed intake data or being able to transform the observed data into a normal distribution. If nonnormal data are not transformed prior to adjustment, or if the applied transformation fails to correct for the nonnormality of the data, then assessments of the prevalence of inadequacy or excess using the adjusted distribution will be inaccurate. Some indication of the importance of this step comes from a closer look at the results of the adjustment procedure applied in the example presented above. Both the mean and the median of the adjusted distribution are slightly lower than the mean and median of the women's 3-day means (Table E-2), suggesting that the adjustment procedure has shifted the original distribution toward 0. This shift is a function of the transformation. Had the transformation more completely achieved the properties of a normal distribution, the observed mean and the adjusted mean would be equivalent.

It may be difficult, if not impossible, to normalize some observed nutrient intake distributions with simple power transformations. Observed distributions of vitamin A, in particular, are notorious for this problem (Aickin and Ritenbaugh, 1991; Beaton et al., 1983). In cases where the data fail to satisfy the assumptions of a normal distribution even when transformed, application of the NRC method and use of the resultant adjusted distribution for nutrient assessment is problematic (Beaton et al., 1997). Depending on the extent of the departure from normality, it may be preferable to not use the data for nutrient assessment. If assessments are conducted on data adjusted without fully satisfying the normality assumption, at minimum, the problem should be noted so that readers can interpret prevalence estimates with greater caution.

Handling Incomplete Data

The NRC method was originally developed for application to data sets with more than one day of intake data per subject. In describing the NRC method here, it has been assumed that an equal number of replicate observations are available for each member of the sample. If there are subjects missing one or more days of intake data, this can be factored into the calculation of $V_{between}$, reducing the denominator of that equation. Nonetheless, it is assumed that few subjects fall into this category.

In large dietary intake surveys it is increasingly common to collect two or more days of intake data on a subsample of the larger sample and use the understanding of within- and between-person variance derived from this subsample to adjust the intake data of the entire sample. (The ISU method [Nusser et al., 1996] is well suited to handling such data.) In surveys involving smaller samples, however, this practice is much less common. The application of estimates of within- and between-person variance from a subsample to the larger sample obviously presumes that the subsample is representative of the larger sample with respect to all characteristics that affect these variance estimates. If starting with a smaller sample, this representativeness may be more difficult to achieve through random sampling. With minor modifications to the NRC method outlined here it is possible to derive variance estimates from a subsample and apply this information to adjust the 1-day intake data for a larger sample. However, given the issue of representativeness, it is preferable to obtain two or more days of intake data on all subjects in a small sample and use all subjects' data in the adjustment procedure.

THE IOWA STATE UNIVERSITY METHOD

Working in conjunction with the U.S. Department of Agriculture, a group of statisticians at ISU developed a method to estimate usual intake distributions from large dietary surveys (Nusser et al., 1996). The method is implemented through a software package called SIDE (Software for Intake Distribution Estimation). It can be used to adjust observed intakes in large dietary surveys as long as two nonconsecutive or three consecutive days of intake data have been collected for a representative subsample of the group. For a full discussion of the ISU method of adjustment, see Guenther and colleagues (1997).

Based on the NRC method, the ISU approach includes a number of statistical enhancements (Guenther et al., 1997). Specifically, the ISU method is designed to transform the intakes for a nutrient to the standard normal distribution, applying procedures that go beyond the simple transformations that analysts can apply in the NRC method. The distribution of usual intakes is then estimated from this distribution of transformed intake values and the estimates are mapped back to the original scale through a bias-adjusted back transformation.

The procedures represent a major advance over the NRC method and a number of other more complicated adjustment procedures that have been proposed (Hoffmann et al., 2002). In addition, the ISU method is designed to take into account other factors such as day of week, time of year, and training or conditioning effects (apparent in patterns of reported intake in relation to the sequence of observations) that may exert systematic effects on the observed distribution of intakes. The ISU method can also account for correlation between observations on consecutive days and for heterogeneous within-person variances (e.g., in cases where the observed level of day-to-day variability in individuals' intakes is directly associated with their mean intake levels). While these refinements could be built into the NRC method, in its simplest form the method does not account for autocorrelation or other systematic effects on within-person variation.

Another particularly valuable feature of the ISU method is its ability to apply sample weighting factors, common in large population surveys, so that the adjusted distribution of intakes truly estimates the distribution of usual intakes in the target population, not just the sample. Thus the ISU method is well suited for use with large survey samples. In a recent evaluation of six different methods, Hoffmann and colleagues (2002) concluded that the ISU method had distinct advantages over the others. Most importantly, the method was applicable across a broad range of normally and nonnormally distributed intakes of food groups and nutrients.

Despite its strengths, however, the ISU method may not be as appropriate as the NRC method for use with small samples. The greater complexity of the ISU method requires a larger sample to ensure that the various steps in the adjustment procedure retain acceptable levels of reliability. A smaller sample can be used with the NRC method because the adjustment procedure is more simplistic (e.g., applying simpler methods of transformation and back-transformation and not accounting for heterogeneity of within-person variance).

OTHER CONSIDERATIONS IN THE APPLICATION OF ADJUSTMENT PROCEDURES

Defining Groups for Data Adjustment

Because nutrient requirements vary by life stage and gender group, assessments of nutrient adequacy are usually conducted separately for particular subgroups of the population. The statistical adjustment of intake data—whether done by the NRC or ISU method—should therefore also be conducted separately for each group for which the nutrient assessment will be conducted. If intake data have been collected across more than one life stage and gender group, it is not appropriate to combine subgroups for the purpose of adjustment and then later subdivide the adjusted data for separate analyses. Similarly, if the intended analysis of nutrient inadequacy is by stratum within a single life stage or gender group (e.g., the assessment of nutrient inadequacy for particular population subgroups defined by income or education levels), then the adjustment of intake data should be conducted separately for each stratum.

Adjusting Intake Variables Expressed as Ratios

To assess the macronutrient composition of diets and examine, for example, the proportion of energy derived from saturated fatty acids, it is necessary to examine the distribution of usual intakes for macronutrients expressed as ratios of total energy intake. The adjustment procedures described here can be applied to intakes expressed as nutrient:energy ratios or as nutrient:nutrient ratios. However, the ratio of interest should be computed for each day of intake data first; the observed intakes are then adjusted to estimate the distribution of usual intakes as ratios. For example, it is not appropriate to compute the adjusted distribution of energy and fat separately and then combine these distributions for analytic purposes.

Underlying Assumptions and Limitations of Adjustment Methods

One important difference in application of the two methods described here is that the ISU method of adjustment is typically applied to the distribution of intakes on day one of data collection, whereas the NRC method is applied to multiple-day means. In the design of large dietary surveys it is becoming increasingly common to collect a second day of intake data on only a subsample of the group. The ISU method is then applied to adjust the entire distribution of intakes on day one using the information about within-person variation that is gleaned from the subsample.

In the application of the NRC method to smaller data sets, typically comprising multiple days of intake data for each member of the sample, multiple-day means are used as the basis for adjustment with the underlying assumption that all days have equivalent validity. In data sets where a sequence effect is observed, with reported energy and nutrient intakes declining systematically across multiple days of data collection (Guenther et al., 1997), the adjustment of intakes to day-one data will result in a higher estimate of usual intake than an adjustment based on individuals' multiple-day means. If it can be assumed that intake on day one has been more accurately reported than on subsequent days, then clearly the adjustment to day-one data will yield a less biased estimate of the distribution of usual intakes. Because good methods to establish the validity of self-reported intakes on particular days of data collection are lacking, it is difficult to determine whether day-one data or multiple-day means are better estimates of true intake. Indeed, the answer may differ depending on the particular group under study and the conditions of data collection.

Neither the NRC nor the ISU method of adjustment is capable of addressing problems of systematic bias due to underreporting of intakes. The approaches must assume that individuals have reported their food intake without systematic bias—on day one, at least, for the ISU method, and across all days of data collection for the NRC method. If intakes have been underreported, the adjusted distribution of intakes will be biased by this underreporting.

Irrespective of the method of adjustment applied, it must also be assumed that reported food intakes have been correctly linked to a food composition database that accurately reflects the energy and nutrient content of the food. Systematic errors in the estimation of nutrient levels in foods consumed will bias the estimated distribution of usual intakes. In the case of nutrients for which food composition data are known to be incomplete, analysts must gauge the extent to which reported intakes will be biased. If intake cannot be estimated without substantial error, it is not appropriate to proceed with nutrient assessment.

Despite these limitations, the adjustment of observed distributions of intake for within-person variance to better estimate the distribution of usual intakes in a group represents a critical step in the assessment of nutrient adequacy or excess. In applying the steps in planning diets for groups, as described in this report, the focus is on planning for usual intakes. The assessments of nutrient adequacy and excess that are required to inform the planning process should be conducted on intake data that have been adjusted to provide the best possible estimate of the distribution of usual intakes in the group.

SAMPLE SAS PROGRAM FOR THE NRC METHOD

(Written by G.H. Beaton, University of Toronto, in December 1988 and modified in January 2002)

This program runs an ANOVA, estimates the partitioning of variance, and calculates the between-person, within-person, and total standard deviations (e.g., SDINTER, SDINTRA, and SDTOTAL, respectively) for the data set at hand with these estimates. The program then adjusts the observed distribution of mean intakes to remove remaining effects of within-person variation in intakes. The adjusted data can then be used as input data for the EAR cut-point or full probability assessment (IOM, 2000a). If the original data are transformed to better approximate a normal distribution, this program should be run on the transformed data and the final adjusted data back-transformed prior to the assessment of nutrient adequacy or excess. Note that the adjustments should be made independently for each stratification (e.g., males and females) and should be run on ratios after the ratio has been calculated.

```
***************************************************************
** NOTE: THIS PROGRAM, AS WRITTEN, ASSUMES THAT THE    **
** INPUT DATA SET HAS ONE RECORD FOR EACH DAY OF        **
** INTAKE.  IF MORE THAN ONE DAY OF INTAKE FOR EACH     **
** SUBJECT APPEARS IN A SINGLE RECORD, THE DATA SET     **
** WILL NEED TO BE REORGANIZED BEFORE THE PROGRAM       **
** IS RUN.                                              **
***************************************************************

PROC ANOVA DATA=YOURDATA OUTSTAT=ANOVSTAT;
CLASS SUBJID;
MODEL NUTRIENT=SUBJID;        *<< Change variable name to nutrient of
interest;
DATA PARTIT1;
SET ANOVSTAT;
MS = SS/DF;
MSERROR = MS; MSMODEL = MS;
DFERROR = DF; DFMODEL = DF;
IF _TYPE_ = 'ERROR' THEN MSMODEL = .;
IF _TYPE_ = 'ANOVA' THEN MSERROR = .;
IF _TYPE_ = 'ERROR' THEN DFMODEL = .;
IF _TYPE_ = 'ANOVA' THEN DFERROR = .;
KEEP MSMODEL DFMODEL MSERROR DFERROR;
PROC UNIVARIATE NOPRINT;
```

continued

```
VAR MSMODEL DFMODEL MSERROR DFERROR;
OUTPUT OUT=PARTIT2 MEAN = MSMODEL DFMODEL MSERROR
DFERROR;
DATA PARTIT3;
SET PARTIT2;
MEANREPL = (DFMODEL+DFERROR+1)/(DFMODEL+1);
ERRORDIF = MSMODEL - MSERROR;
IF ERRORDIF LT 0 THEN ERRORDIF = 0;
SDINTRA = MSERROR**0.5;
SDINTER = (ERRORDIF / MEANREPL)**0.5;
SDTOTAL = (SDINTER**2 +(SDINTRA**2/MEANREPL))**0.5;
INDEX=1;
KEEP SDINTER SDTOTAL INDEX;
PROC MEANS NOPRINT DATA=YOURDATA;
  VAR NUTRIENT; BY SUBJID;
   OUTPUT OUT=SUBJMEAN MEAN=SMEAN;
DATA SUBJMEAN; SET SUBJMEAN; INDEX=1;
PROC UNIVARIATE NOPRINT; VAR SMEAN;
OUTPUT OUT=MEANS  MEAN = GMEAN;
DATA MEANS; SET MEANS; INDEX=1;
DATA ADJUST;
MERGE SUBJMEAN PARTIT3 MEANS;
BY INDEX;
NRCADJ = GMEAN + (SMEAN - GMEAN) * SDINTER/SDTOTAL;
KEEP SUBJID NRCADJ;
RUN;


****************************************
** THIS IS NOW THE ADJUSTED      **
** DATA TO BE USED IN ANALYSIS   **
** NEED TO DO FOR EACH OF THE    **
** INTAKE VARIABLES IF THIS      **
** PROCEDURE IS TO BE EMPLOYED   **
****************************************


DATA FINAL; MERGE YOURDATA ADJUST; BY SUBJID;
PROC PRINT;
TITLE 'NUTRIENT DATA SHOWING INDIVIDUAL OBS, MEAN, NRC
ADJUSTED';
RUN;
```

F
Biographical Sketches of Subcommittee Members

SUSAN I. BARR, Ph.D., R.D.N. (*chair*) is a professor of nutrition at the University of British Columbia. Her research interests focus on the associations among nutrition, physical activity, and bone health in women, and she has authored over 80 publications. Dr. Barr served as vice president of the Canadian Dietetic Association (now Dietitians of Canada) and is a fellow of both the Dietitians of Canada and the American College of Sports Medicine. She also holds memberships in the American Dietetic Association and the American Society for Nutritional Sciences. She is currently a member of the Scientific Advisory Board of the Osteoporosis Society of Canada, the Health Canada Expert Advisory Committee on Dietary Reference Intakes, and the Board of Trustees of the National Institute of Nutrition. She serves as a member of the Board of Editors for the *International Journal of Sport Nutrition and Exercise Metabolism* and *Nutrition Today*. Dr. Barr received a Ph.D. in human nutrition from the University of Minnesota and is a registered dietitian in Canada.

TANYA D. AGURS-COLLINS, Ph.D., R.D. is an associate professor in the Department of Medicine, Howard University College of Medicine and a nutritional epidemiologist in the Division of Cancer Prevention, Control and Population Science, Howard University Cancer Center in Washington, D.C. Her primary research interests include nutrition and cancer prevention in minority populations. Dr. Agurs-Collins has worked at the D.C. Office on Aging as nutrition program manager and was president of the District of Columbia Metropolitan Area Dietetic Association. She was a member of the mayoral-appointed Board of Dietetics and Nutrition of the District of Columbia Government and the recipient of the Outstanding Dietitian of the Year Award, District of Columbia Metropolitan Area Dietetic Association. She earned her Ph.D. in nutrition from the Pennsylvania State University.

ALICIA L. CARRIQUIRY, Ph.D. is a professor in the Department of Statistics and an associate provost at Iowa State University. Since 1990 Dr. Carriquiry collaborated with scientists from the U.S. Department of Agriculture (USDA), the U.S. Environmental Protection Agency, and the U.S. Department of Health and Human Services. She is a consultant for ABT Associates, Environcorp, Kemin International, and Mathematica Policy Research, and is an affiliate for the Law and Economics Consulting Group. At present, Dr. Carriquiry is investigating the statistical issues associated with estimating usual nutrient intake distributions by combining food and supplement sources, and she recently completed reports on improving USDA's food intake surveys and methods to estimate adjusted intake, and biochemical measurement distributions for the Third National Health and Nutrition Examination Survey. Dr. Carriquiry is the current past president of the International Society for Bayesian Analysis and is an elected member of the International Statistical Institute. She is editor of *Statistical Science* and serves on the Executive Committee of the Board of Directors of the National Institute of Statistical Science and of the Institute of Mathematical Statistics. She was elected fellow of the American Statistical Association in 1999. She currently serves on a National Research Council panel and on another National Academy of Sciences committee. Dr. Carriquiry's research interests include nutrition and dietary assessment, Bayesian methods and applications, mixed models and variance component estimation, environmental statistics, stochastic volatility, and linear and nonlinear filtering. She received her Ph.D. in statistics and animal science from Iowa State.

ANN M. COULSTON, M.S., R.D., F.A.D.A. is an established expert in clinical nutrition and research. She is a partner at Hattner/Coulston Nutrition Associates, LLC where she serves as a nutrition consultant to public relation firms and the food and nutrition industry. She is also a nutrition consultant at Stanford University School of Medicine. She is a past president of the American Dietetic Association (ADA) and of the California Dietetic Association. She spent more than 20 years performing clinical research at Stanford University that centered on the nutritional needs of adults and the elderly. Her special research interest is in the nutritional management of diabetes and dyslipidemias, particularly in the role of dietary carbohydrates. Ms. Coulston has been recognized by the ADA Foundation for Excellence in the practice of clinical nutrition and research and has also received the ADA's Medallion Award for leadership and the Distinguished Service and Outstanding Member Award of the California Dietetic Association.

BARBARA L. DEVANEY, Ph.D. is an economist and senior fellow at Mathematica Policy Research in Princeton, New Jersey. Her substantive expertise is in the areas of food assistance and nutrition policy and maternal and child health policy and programs. She has designed and conducted several studies of the school nutrition programs, the Food Stamp Program, and the WIC program. She received her Ph.D. in economics at the University of Michigan.

JANET R. HUNT, Ph.D., R.D is a scientist and research leader at the U.S. Department of Agriculture/Agricultural Research Service (USDA/ARS) Human Nutrition Research Center in Grand Forks, North Dakota. She is also an adjunct professor of nutrition and dietetics at the University of North Dakota. Dr. Hunt's responsibilities at USDA/ARS include leading the Mineral Utilization Research Management Unit and conducting research on human trace element requirements and dietary bioavailability. She has extensively published on the topics of iron and zinc absorption and iron status. Dr. Hunt serves on the editorial board for the *Journal of the American Dietetic Association* and co-authored the association's Position Statement on Vitamin and Mineral Supplements. She is also a member of the American Society for Clinical Nutrition and the American Society for Nutritional Sciences. Dr. Hunt received her Ph.D. in nutrition from the University of Minnesota.

SUZANNE P. MURPHY, Ph.D., R.D. is a researcher at the Cancer Research Center of Hawaii at the University of Hawaii, Honolulu. Previously she was an adjunct associate professor in the Department of Nutritional Sciences at the University of California at Berkeley and director of the California Expanded Food and Nutrition Program at the University of California at Davis. Dr. Murphy's research interests include dietary assessment methodology, development of food composition databases, and nutritional epidemiology. She served as a member of the National Nutrition Monitoring Advisory Council and the 2000 Dietary Guidelines Advisory Committee, and is currently on editorial boards for the *Journal of Food Composition and Analysis* and *Nutrition Today*. Dr. Murphy is a member of numerous professional organizations including the American Dietetic Association, the American Society for Nutritional Sciences, the American Public Health Association, the American Society for Clinical Nutrition, and the Society for Nutrition Education. She has over 50 publications on dietary assessment methodology and has lectured nationally and internationally on this subject. She received her B.S. in mathematics from Temple University and her Ph.D. in nutrition from the University of California at Berkeley.

VALERIE TARASUK, Ph.D. is an associate professor of the Faculty of Medicine at the University of Toronto's Department of Nutritional Sciences and Public Health Sciences. Her primary research interests are in domestic food insecurity, food policy, and dietary assessment. Dr. Tarasuk has served on several committees and advisory groups including the Nutrition Expert Advisory Group of the Canadian Community Health Survey and the External Advisory Panel for Food Directorate Review of Policies on the Addition of Vitamins and Minerals to Foods. She chaired the Data Review Panels for the Prince Edward Island and Saskatchewan Nutrition Surveys. Dr. Tarasuk is currently a member of Health Canada's Expert Advisory Committee on Dietary Reference Intakes and the Institute of Medicine Committee on the Use of Dietary Reference Intakes in Nutrition Labeling. She earned her Ph.D. in nutritional sciences at the University of Toronto.

DRI Committee Liaison

WILLIAM M. RAND, Ph.D. is a professor of biostatistics in the Department of Family Medicine and Community Health, Tufts University School of Medicine and also is a professor at the Tufts Schools of Veterinary Medicine and of Dental Medicine. Prior to his appointment at Tufts he was in the Nutrition and Food Science Department at the Massachusetts Institute of Technology (MIT). While at MIT he helped develop and served as the first director of INFOODS (International Network of Food Data Systems), and managed the United Nations University research efforts in the area of protein requirements. He was a member of the 1981 Food and Agriculture Organization/World Health Organization/United Nations University (FAO/WHO/UNU) Consultation of Energy and Protein Requirements, and is a member of the current FAO/WHO/UNU Consultation on Protein and Amino Acid Requirements. Dr. Rand's general expertise is in multivariate statistical modeling and application of statistics to biomedical problems. He received his Ph.D. in biostatistics from the University of California at Los Angeles.

Index

A

Acceptable Macronutrient Range, 30, 78, 80

Adequacy of nutrient intake. *See also* Prevalence of inadequate intakes
assessment of, 95-96, 196; *see also* Dietary assessment
confidence levels, 84, 94
criteria of, 23, 24, 28, 29, 30, 83, 102, 166
energy intake and, 31-32, 91
in group-level planning, 29, 75, 81, 83, 91, 95-96, 114, 115, 184, 185
in individual-level planning, 26, 37, 45-47, 50, 53
observed difference and, 37
probability of correct conclusion about, 37, 81
quantitative assessments of, 37
risk-reduction based indicator of, 22, 23
uncertainty in, 29

Adequate Intakes (AIs). *See also specific nutrients*
applicable population, 25
context for use, 4, 23, 39
Daily Values on food labels compared, 52
defined, 3, 24-25, 39
derivation of, 22-23, 25, 39, 83

EARs compared, 4, 25, 154
and food guides, 47, 49
in group-level planning, 9, 11-12, 83-84, 85-87, 94-95, 103
and group mean intake, 83, 84, 85-87
in individual-level planning, 4, 6, 35, 37, 39, 41
menu planning with, 11-12, 83-84, 85-87
and nutrient density approaches, 94, 103
nutrients, by life-stage group, 85-87
and prevalence of inadequate intakes, 84, 94
RDAs compared, 4, 25
replacement with EARs and RDAs, 25, 154
research recommendations, 25, 154
uncertainty in, 4, 39, 133-134
uses, 2, 4, 25

Adjusting intake distributions
backtransformation of adjusted data, 166, 200-201, 203
defining groups for, 204
EAR and, 65-68
EAR cut-point method and, 10, 109, 201
energy, 33, 205
estimation of within- and between-person variance, 33, 63-64, 199-200, 204, 207-208

213

SUMMARY TABLE 1 Dietary Reference Intakes (DRIs):
Estimated Average Requirements for Groups
Food and Nutrition Board, Institute of Medicine,
National Academies

Life Stage Group	Carbo-hydrate (g/d)	Protein (g/d)	Vit A (µg/d)[a]	Vit C (mg/d)	Vit E (mg/d)[b]	Thiamin (mg/d)
Infants						
7–12 mo		10				
Children						
1–3 y	100	11	210	13	5	0.4
4–8 y	100	15	275	22	6	0.5
Males						
9–13 y	100	27	445	39	9	0.7
14–18 y	100	44	630	63	12	1.0
19–30 y	100	46	625	75	12	1.0
31–50 y	100	46	625	75	12	1.0
51–70 y	100	46	625	75	12	1.0
> 70 y	100	46	625	75	12	1.0
Females						
9–13 y	100	28	420	39	9	0.7
14–18 y	100	38	485	56	12	0.9
19–30 y	100	38	500	60	12	0.9
31–50 y	100	38	500	60	12	0.9
51–70 y	100	38	500	60	12	0.9
> 70 y	100	38	500	60	12	0.9
Pregnancy						
≤ 18 y	135	50	530	66	12	1.2
19–30 y	135	50	550	70	12	1.2
31–50 y	135	50	550	70	12	1.2
Lactation						
≤ 18 y	160	60	880	96	16	1.2
19–30 y	160	60	900	100	16	1.2
31–50 y	160	60	900	100	16	1.2

continued

NOTE: This table presents Estimated Average Requirements (EARs), which serve three purposes: for assessing adequacy of population intakes, for planning the adequacy of population intakes, and as the basis for calculating Recommended Dietary Allowances (RDAs) for individuals for those nutrients. EARs have not been established for vitamin D, vitamin K, pantothenic acid, biotin, choline, calcium, chromium, fluoride, manganese, or other nutrients not yet evaluated via the DRI process.

[a] As retinol activity equivalents (RAEs). 1 RAE = 1 µg retinol, 12 µg β-carotene, 24 µg α-carotene, or 24 µg β-cryptoxanthin. The RAE for dietary provitamin A carotenoids is two-fold greater than retinol equivalents (RE), whereas the RAE for preformed vitamin A is the same as RE.

(DRIs): Estimated Average Requirements for Groups
Food and Nutrition Board, Institute of Medicine,
National Academies

Life Stage Group	Ribo-flavin (mg/d)	Niacin (mg/d)[c]	Vit B6 (mg/d)	Folate (µg/d)[a]	Vit B12 (µg/d)	Copper (µg/d)
Infants						
7–12 mo						
Children						
1–3 y	0.4	5	0.4	120	0.7	260
4–8 y	0.5	6	0.5	160	1.0	340
Males						
9–13 y	0.8	9	0.8	250	1.5	540
14–18 y	1.1	12	1.1	330	2.0	685
19–30 y	1.1	12	1.1	320	2.0	700
31–50 y	1.1	12	1.1	320	2.0	700
51–70 y	1.1	12	1.4	320	2.0	700
> 70 y	1.1	12	1.4	320	2.0	700
Females						
9–13 y	0.8	9	0.8	250	1.5	540
14–18 y	0.9	11	1.0	330	2.0	685
19–30 y	0.9	11	1.1	320	2.0	700
31–50 y	0.9	11	1.1	320	2.0	700
51–70 y	0.9	11	1.3	320	2.0	700
> 70 y	0.9	11	1.3	320	2.0	700
Pregnancy						
≤ 18 y	1.2	14	1.6	520	2.2	785
19–30 y	1.2	14	1.6	520	2.2	800
31–50 y	1.2	14	1.6	520	2.2	800
Lactation						
≤ 18 y	1.3	13	1.7	450	2.4	985
19–30 y	1.3	13	1.7	450	2.4	1,000
31–50 y	1.3	13	1.7	450	2.4	1,000

[b] As α-tocopherol. α-Tocopherol includes *RRR*-α-tocopherol, the only form of α-tocopherol that occurs naturally in foods, and the *2R*-stereoisomeric forms of α-tocopherol (*RRR*-, *RSR*-, *RRS*-, and *RSS*-α-tocopherol) that occur in fortified foods and supplements. It does not include the *2S*-stereoisomeric forms of α-tocopherol (*SRR*-, *SSR*-, *SRS*-, and *SSS*-α-tocopherol), also found in fortified foods and supplements.

[c] As niacin equivalents (NE). 1 mg of niacin = 60 mg of tryptophan.

[d] As dietary folate equivalents (DFE). 1 DFE = 1 µg food folate = 0.6 µg of folic acid from fortified food or as a supplement consumed with food = 0.5 µg of a supplement taken on an empty stomach.

Iodine (μg/d)	Iron (mg/d)	Magnesium (mg/d)	Molybdenum (μg/d)	Phosphorus (mg/d)	Selenium (μg/d)	Zinc (mg/d)
	6.9					2.5
65	3.0	65	13	380	17	2.5
65	4.1	110	17	405	23	4.0
73	5.9	200	26	1,055	35	7.0
95	7.7	340	33	1,055	45	8.5
95	6	330	34	580	45	9.4
95	6	350	34	580	45	9.4
95	6	350	34	580	45	9.4
95	6	350	34	580	45	9.4
73	5.7	200	26	1,055	35	7.0
95	7.9	300	33	1,055	45	7.3
95	8.1	255	34	580	45	6.8
95	8.1	265	34	580	45	6.8
95	5	265	34	580	45	6.8
95	5	265	34	580	45	6.8
160	23	335	40	1,055	49	10.5
160	22	290	40	580	49	9.5
160	22	300	40	580	49	9.5
209	7	300	35	1,055	59	10.9
209	6.5	255	36	580	59	10.4
209	6.5	265	36	580	59	10.4

SOURCES: *Dietary Reference Intakes for Calcium, Phosphorous, Magnesium, Vitamin D, and Fluoride* (1997); *Dietary Reference Intakes for Thiamin, Riboflavin, Niacin, Vitamin B6, Folate, Vitamin B12, Pantothenic Acid, Biotin, and Choline* (1998); *Dietary Reference Intakes for Vitamin C, Vitamin E, Selenium, and Carotenoids* (2000); *Dietary Reference Intakes for Vitamin A, Vitamin K, Arsenic, Boron, Chromium, Copper, Iodine, Iron, Manganese, Molybdenum, Nickel, Silicon, Vanadium, and Zinc* (2001); and *Dietary Reference Intakes for Energy, Carbohydrate, Fiber, Fat, Fatty Acids, Cholesterol, Protein, and Amino Acids* (2002). These reports may be accessed via www.nap.edu.

SUMMARY TABLE 2 Dietary Reference Intakes (DRIs): Tolerable Upper Intake Levels (UL[a]), Vitamins Food and Nutrition Board, Institute of Medicine, National Academies

Life Stage Group	Vitamin A (µg/d)[b]	Vitamin C (mg/d)	Vitamin D (µg/d)	Vitamin E (mg/d)[c,d]
Infants				
0–6 mo	600	ND[f]	25	ND
7–12 mo	600	ND	25	ND
Children				
1–3 y	600	400	50	200
4–8 y	900	650	50	300
Males, Females				
9–13 y	1,700	1,200	50	600
14–18 y	2,800	1,800	50	800
19–70 y	3,000	2,000	50	1,000
> 70 y	3,000	2,000	50	1,000
Pregnancy				
≤ 18 y	2,800	1,800	50	800
19–50 y	3,000	2,000	50	1,000
Lactation				
≤ 18 y	2,800	1,800	50	800
19–50 y	3,000	2,000	50	1,000

[a] UL = The maximum level of daily nutrient intake that is likely to pose no risk of adverse effects. Unless otherwise specified, the UL represents total intake from food, water, and supplements. Due to lack of suitable data, ULs could not be established for vitamin K, thiamin, riboflavin, vitamin B_{12}, pantothenic acid, biotin, or carotenoids. In the absence of ULs, extra caution may be warranted in consuming levels above recommended intakes.

[b] As preformed vitamin A only.

[c] As α-tocopherol; applies to any form of supplemental α-tocopherol.

[d] The ULs for vitamin E, niacin, and folate apply to synthetic forms obtained from supplements, fortified foods, or a combination of the two.

[e] β-Carotene supplements are advised only to serve as a provitamin A source for individuals at risk of vitamin A deficiency.

232

Vitamin K	Thiamin	Ribo-flavin	Niacin $(mg/d)^d$	Vitamin B_6 (mg/d)	Folate $(\mu g/d)^d$
ND	ND	ND	ND	ND	ND
ND	ND	ND	ND	ND	ND
ND	ND	ND	10	30	300
ND	ND	ND	15	40	400
ND	ND	ND	20	60	600
ND	ND	ND	30	80	800
ND	ND	ND	35	100	1,000
ND	ND	ND	35	100	1,000
ND	ND	ND	30	80	800
ND	ND ·	ND	35	100	1,000
ND	ND	ND	30	80	800
ND	ND	ND	35	100	1,000

continued

f ND = Not determinable due to lack of data of adverse effects in this age group and concern with regard to lack of ability to handle excess amounts. Source of intake should be from food only to prevent high levels of intake.

SOURCES: *Dietary Reference Intakes for Calcium, Phosphorous, Magnesium, Vitamin D, and Fluoride* (1997); *Dietary Reference Intakes for Thiamin, Riboflavin, Niacin, Vitamin B_6, Folate, Vitamin B_{12}, Pantothenic Acid, Biotin, and Choline* (1998); *Dietary Reference Intakes for Vitamin C, Vitamine E, Selenium, and Carotenoids* (2000); and *Dietary Reference Intakes for Vitamin A, Vitamin K, Arsenic, Boron, Chromium, Copper, Iodine, Iron, Manganese, Molybdenum, Nickel, Silicon, Vanadium, and Zinc* (2001). These reports may be accessed via www.nap.edu.

(DRIs): Tolerable Upper Intake Levels (UL^a), Vitamins
Food and Nutrition Board, Institute of Medicine,
National Academies

Life Stage Group	Vitamin B$_{12}$	Pantothenic Acid	Biotin	Choline (g/d)	Carotenoids^e
Infants					
0–6 mo	ND	ND	ND	ND	ND
7–12 mo	ND	ND	ND	ND	ND
Children					
1–3 y	ND	ND	ND	1.0	ND
4–8 y	ND	ND	ND	1.0	ND
Males, Females					
9–13 y	ND	ND	ND	2.0	ND
14–18 y	ND	ND	ND	3.0	ND
19–70 y	ND	ND	ND	3.5	ND
> 70 y	ND	ND	ND	3.5	ND
Pregnancy					
≤ 18 y	ND	ND	ND	3.0	ND
19–50 y	ND	ND	ND	3.5	ND
Lactation					
≤ 18 y	ND	ND	ND	3.0	ND
19–50 y	ND	ND	ND	3.5	ND